HEALTH
PROMOTION
FOR THE
ELDERLY

Colleen Keller / Julie Fleury

Sage Publications, Inc.
International Educational and Professional Publisher
Thousand Oaks ■ London ■ New Delhi

For information:

Sage Publications, Inc.
2455 Teller Road
Thousand Oaks, California 91320
E-mail: order@sagepub.com

Sage Publications Ltd.
6 Bonhill Street
London EC2A 4PU
United Kingdom

Sage Publications India Pvt. Ltd.
M-32 Market
Greater Kailash I
New Delhi 110 048 India

Printed in the United States of America

Library of Congress Cataloging-in-Publication Data

Keller, Colleen, 1949–
    Health promotion for the elderly / by Colleen Keller and Julie Fleury.
        p.   cm.
    Includes bibliographical references and index.
    ISBN 0-7619-1473-0 (cloth: acid-free paper)
    ISBN 0-7619-1474-9 (pbk.: acid-free paper)
    1. Aged—Health and hygiene.   2. Health promotion.
    I. Fleury, Julie.   II. Title.
    RA564.8 K438   2000
    613'.0438—dc21   99-050430

This book is printed on acid-free paper.

00   01   02   03   04   05   06   7   6   5   4   3   2   1

Acquiring Editor:	Jim Nageotte
Editorial Assistant:	Anna Howland
Production Editor:	Wendy Westgate
Editorial Assistant:	Victoria Cheng
Typesetter:	Lynn Miyata
Cover Designer:	Candice Harman
Indexer:	Molly Hall

Contents

Preface

This text is the result of 2 years of the development of the state of the science regarding health promotion issues for older people. Special emphasis has been placed on vulnerable groups, including the minority elderly and women, and on modifiable risk factors for chronic illness and debilitation in older people, such as smoking, obesity, and sedentary lifestyles. The content is organized to delineate clearly the health risks of the elderly and health promotion efforts for the elderly. What we have presented is the state of the science in terms of what is known about risks in the elderly and what is known about the efficacy of interventions in health promotion for the elderly. We have included information concerning the health issues relevant to minorities, including the issue of poverty. We have discussed theoretical models employed in the development of health promotion interventions, their merits and weaknesses. In addition, the issue of community-based intervention models and community empowerment for the elderly is discussed. These elements are not included in other health promotion texts, and they represent a significant strength in this one. We have discussed issues surrounding vitamin supplementation, use of alternative supplements for hormone replacement, and the issue of cardiovascular risk reduction in the older person. These are issues on which the clinician needs timely and relevant information.

CHAPTER 1

Changes Accompanying Aging and Functional Assessment

The importance of health for all, both young and old, across the life span has long been emphasized as a significant societal goal. Given the growth in the human population and our effects on one another and the environment, the health and well-being of any group increasingly depends on the health and well-being of all. A 65-year-old man living today can expect to live another 14.8 years; for a 65-year-old woman, life expectancy is another 19 years (Census Bureau, 1990). These long periods of life after age 65 provide the opportunity for health promotion efforts in older people. Thus, health promotion efforts should not only address strategies to decrease the sequelae of chronic and debilitating conditions but also improve functional ability and quality of life in this group of people.

Since the beginning of the twentieth century, significant changes have occurred in the size, age structure, health profile, and health care use patterns of the U.S. population (Furner, Brody, & Jankowski, 1997). Overall, the size of the population has more than tripled. The population has aged; persons 65 years of age and over currently make up almost 13% of the total population, more than three times that seen in 1900. More than 70% of the population now live to age 65 (Neugarten & Reed, 1997). Furthermore, more than 30% survive to be 80 years of age and over (Brody, Brock, & Williams, 1987). A significant aspect of the population change has been the shift in the age composition, with the population 65 years and older increasing at a rate more than twice that of the total population (Verbrugge, 1989). For those between 65

1

and 74 years of age, mortality rates from all causes fell by 35.6% over the past 4 decades (National Center for Health Statistics, 1997). There are also indications that the elderly population is itself aging; significant expansion in the population aged 85 and over has been noted (Furner et al., 1997). For those 75 to 84 years of age, mortality rates from all causes have decreased by 36.9% over the past 40 years, and for those 85 or older, decreases in mortality were 25.5% (National Center for Health Statistics, 1997).

The current aging of the population is projected to continue into the twenty-first century (Furner et al., 1997). Although the population 65 years of age and older will equal 13% of the total population in the year 2000, projections from the Census Bureau indicate that the older population will number 87 million, 23% of the total population, by the year 2050 (Census Bureau, 1990). The projected expansion of the older population is greatest among the oldest old, those persons 85 years of age and over. This group will number 5 million in the year 2000 and is expected to increase approximately threefold by the year 2040 (Census Bureau, 1990). The population of elderly minorities is projected to increase dramatically. For example, African American elderly are expected to increase by 150% over the next 40 years, Native American elderly by 200%, and Hispanic and Asian Americans by 200% (Markides & Miranda, 1997).

The dramatic increase in the elderly population, both presently and in the future, must direct our efforts toward understanding and promoting the health and well-being of these individuals and communities. Clearly, the implications of age-related demographic changes for our society and health care systems are great. Although recent studies suggest that chronic illness and disability rates among older people have decreased, for many older people, age is equated with multiple illnesses, disability, and a reduced quality of life. The primary aim of this chapter is to examine the complex relations among lifestyle patterns, social constructs and issues, and health promotion efforts in the aging population. Medical technology and improved lifestyles have added years to the lives of many. However, health care providers continue to face the challenge of promoting health, independence, and well-being within these years.

GOALS FOR HEALTH PROMOTION IN OLDER PEOPLE

Health promotion and disease prevention efforts are categorized as primary, secondary, or tertiary. Primary prevention refers to those activities that reduce the risk for the development of a disease process or illness. Secondary prevention is directed toward the early detection of a disease process, usually before it becomes clinically evident. Tertiary prevention is directed toward the reduction of disability related to disease processes. All three stages of health promotion and prevention are affected by significant lifestyle behaviors, such as cigarette smoking, sedentary activity, and inadequate nutritional practice.

Our knowledge base concerning the potential role for primary and secondary prevention in older people remains relatively small. However, behavioral, social, psychological, and socioenvironmental factors appear to play an important role in the health of aged persons. These factors may become increasingly important in older age and may represent critical areas of intervention in primary health care and public health practice. Although longevity has increased for the population at large, quality of life, particularly in the later years, has not necessarily increased. Chronic illness, frailty, and a reduced quality of life frequently characterize old age, particularly for the oldest old (see Table 1.1). It is essential to consider the role of health promotion and risk reduction behaviors across the life span to maintain productivity to older age.

Both the cost of health care and the number of older adults using this care are increasing rapidly. The percentage of national resources spent on health care services in the United States currently surpasses that of all other countries. Older adults consume the majority of medical services and prescription medications in the United States, so health promotion efforts directed toward older people have a potentially large impact. Similarly, a high percentage of older adults suffer from one or more chronic illnesses that require costly medical treatment.

Given the increasing numbers of older adults, the potential burden of subclinical disease and comorbidity—which often accompany aging—and the increased potential for impaired function and decreased quality of life, clinicians and other health care providers must direct new and more effective approaches to health promotion among the aged. The need to prevent the development of disease and to lengthen years of productive life must be considered when exploring health promotion approaches for older people. As subclinical disease begins to develop, health promotion approaches are directed toward reducing the rate of debilitation and delaying the onset of chronic illness and loss of independence. These preventive efforts must target effective primary care, which includes patient risk assessment and early intervention. Primary screening and risk assessment also must include a risk reduction emphasis to decrease or ameliorate the rate of disease progression. Reduction or delay in disease progression will help to limit the development of functional

TABLE 1.1   Summary of Age-Related Changes and Sequelae

Age-Related Changes	Sequelae
PULMONARY SYSTEM	
Loss of pulmonary reserve, increased stiffness of chest wall, diminished muscle strength	Reduced maximal inspiratory/expiratory force
Loss of elastic recoil, alveoli thin and enlarged	Reduced surface area for gas exchange Increased residual volume
CARDIOVASCULAR SYSTEM	
Valves thicken and stiffen	Reduced contractility
Decrease in left ventricular compliance	Reduced maximal heart rate and reduced aerobic capacity
Aortic and arterial thickness	Increased systolic pressure
Decreased myocardial function	Decreased stroke volume
INTEGUMENTARY SYSTEM	
Loss of subcutaneous fat	Cold/heat intolerance
20% decrease in dermis	Cold/heat intolerance
10%-20% decrease in melanocytes	Inability to protect self from ultraviolet rays
Reduction in capillary network	Skin atrophy, decreased rate of healing
Inadequate support for cutaneous blood vessels	Purpuric lesions
MUSCULOSKELETAL SYSTEM	
Decrease in bone strength	Risk of fractures
Decrease in lean and fat mass	Increase in unfavorable fat distribution
10%-40% decrease in muscle strength	Slower movement/difficult mobility
Decrease in size and number of muscle fibers	Decreased isometric strength
Decline in joint function	Difficult mobility
NERVOUS SYSTEM	
Generalized slowing and wasting of nervous system	Slower reaction time, vertigo, and gait disturbances
ENDOCRINE SYSTEM	
Decreases in glucose tolerance, reduced estrogen secretion	Alteration on regional body fat to less favorable distribution; increase in unfavorable blood lipids, increased risk of bone density reduction

impairment, including physical, cognitive, social, or psychological sequelae (Kaplan, 1997).

IDENTIFICATION OF CHANGES ACCOMPANYING AGING

Aging is not a disease but the normal course of the human condition. Prevention of aging is neither desirable nor realistic. However, promotion of health and prevention of chronic illness and disability are significant goals for older people. Our entire view of aging has been distorted by equating it with disease and disuse. In current times, virtually no one lives long enough to die of "natural causes." Rather, people die from conditions that are largely preventable given available knowledge. It is important to recognize that aging processes are gradual and continuous and form a progression of changes, some orderly and predictable and others unpredictable. Social as well as biological timetables govern the sequence of change (Kaplan, 1997).

Human aging is a variable and individual process, which may best be examined as part of the life trajectory (Neugarten & Neugarten, 1986). Thus, old age is not a separable period of life but a gradual and progressive process, which reflects historical interests, relationships, and lifestyle behaviors. Although aging frequently is marked by reduced physiologic capacity, the manifestations of aging also may be determined by genetic and lifestyle influences (Baker & Martin, 1997). Aging itself is not a disease to be prevented but a normal part of the human condition. For many, older adulthood reflects vigor, productivity, and well-being. However, for others, chronic illness, dependence, and despair mark the aging process (Neugarten & Reed, 1997). Although it is true that as individuals age, they are at greater risk of developing chronic health problems such as arthritis, cardiovascular disease, diabetes, and sensory impairments, these conditions are not inherent in the aging process. This distinction between normal aging and disease is important for health care providers to be able to recognize for the purposes of diagnosis and treatment. Much of the focus on aging has been as a deterioration process and on older adults as frail and dependent, rather than on healthy aging leading to an active and independent old age.

A life cycle perspective of aging has important implications for health planners and providers (Neugarten & Reed, 1997). Except for retirement, old age is not a separable period of life. The aging process is neither abrupt in its onset nor, for most persons, marked by dramatic changes in interests, personal commitments, or, until a major change in health occurs, in lifestyle. The individual's social and health characteristics in old age are, in large part, the outcomes of earlier lifestyles and earlier health histories.

There are wide individual differences in the physiological response to aging as well as differences in the rates of aging. These vary tremendously in the rates in which they occur, both from person to person and in the same person, from one bodily system or psychological function to another. As noted previously, aging processes are gradual and continuous and form a progression of changes, some orderly and predictable and others unpredictable. Social as well as biological timetables govern the sequence of change (Baker & Martin, 1997). There are wide individual differences in reactions to aging as well as differences in the rates of aging. These vary tremendously in the rates in which they occur, both from person to person and within the same person, from one bodily system or psychological function to another.

The rate of aging is determined in part by genetic factors and in part by the individual's behavior that can compensate for or accelerate the aging process. For example, in many cases, habits such as cigarette smoking, inactivity, and poor diet can increase the individual's vulnerability to disease or the effects of aging. For many individuals, age-related changes may contribute to psychological distress. Although these changes may not be reversible, compensatory measures can be taken to improve emotional well-being. Taking advantage of the "use it or lose it" principle, such as involvement in physical activity and other attempts to maintain functioning, can help slow or offset the physical and psychological consequences of aging.

There is no single metabolic, genetic, or chemical trigger that contributes to the gradual decline in body systems and organs (Hickey, Speers, & Prohaska, 1997). Both the pathology of disease and the aging process appear to be a series of complex and diverse time- and age-related changes. It is less important to make a distinction between disease pathology and age-related changes than it is to have an understanding of the interrelation of the two processes. First, age-related changes and the pathology of disease differ in the individual's response to them. For example, age-related changes might not "cause" disease but may lead to altered susceptibility to disease (Hickey et al., 1997). Second, some age-related changes—for example, sensory-neurological-perceptive changes—may alter the individual's response to clinical warning signs, such as precancerous lesions (Hickey et al., 1997). Third, environmental stresses, including psychological and social stresses, may predispose older people to pathology not evident in those individuals less susceptible to environmental stress.

In spite of the within- and between-individual variation in age-related changes, there are some salient characteristics hallmarking aging that are common and visible. A brief overview of the common and visible age-related changes follows; the reduction of risk and pathology related to these changes are targeted in health promotion and prevention efforts.

Integumentary System

The most salient and visible aspect of the aging body is the skin. Thus, changes in the skin are perhaps the most obvious reflection of the aging process. Although overall epidermal thinning is noted in aging skin, areas of the epidermis may thicken in response to extrinsic factors, such as chronic exposure to sunlight. The skin loses about 20% of its thickness, giving the appearance of transparency and thinness (Goldfarb, Ellis, & Yoorless, 1997). There is loss of underlying subcutaneous tissue, contributing to the perception of older people of thermal cold (Goldfarb et al., 1997). With advancing age, the cells of the inner layer of the epidermis may demonstrate a more random arrangement and slower reproduction compared with younger people, with greater variation in nuclear and cytoplasmic size (Matteson, 1997). Melanocytes in the basal layer of the epidermis may decrease in number, causing aging skin to appear pale.

The dermis, significantly affected by elements such as the sun, also undergoes intrinsic changes (Goldfarb et al., 1997). These changes are related to the aging process that reflects genetic tendencies accompanied by dermal thinning, loss of elasticity, and the deepening of expression lines. The major morphological changes include wrinkling, laxity, uneven pigmentation, and proliferative lesions (Dalziel & Bickers, 1992).

Age-related changes are complicated by the fact that the skin is subject to repeated and cumulative environmental damage (Dalziel & Bickers, 1992). Many of the changes assumed to be due to intrinsic aging processes are as a result of repeated exposure to physical elements. Therefore, protecting skin from the environment can prevent many of the aging effects previously thought to be unavoidable. Exposure to sunlight is thought to have the most damaging effects. Ultraviolet B light is most responsible for chronic damage from the sun and ultraviolet A light less so (Goldfarb et al., 1997). The degree of photoaging varies not only with solar exposure but also with the individual. Melanin pigment is protective against the sun's effect, so a fair-skinned person is more susceptible to sun damage than someone with greater pigmentation.

The processes that underlie age-related integumentary changes also have a negative effect on the protective function of the skin. There is a decrease in the vascularity of the dermal skin and greater vascular fragility (Gilchrest &

Yaar, 1992; Leydon, 1990; Lober & Fenske, 1990). There is a noted decrease in vascular responsiveness, evidenced by decreasing numbers of epithelial cells and blood vessels (Matteson, 1997). Compromised vessels have a reduced healing capability with age, resulting in greater risk for decubitus ulcers and prolonged wound closure. Compromised thermoregulation predisposes older people to heat stroke and hypothermia, primarily due to reduced vasodilatation or vasoconstriction of dermal arterioles and decreased subcutaneous fat tissue. Age-related changes in skin and subcutaneous fat structure predispose the older individual to cold intolerance, dry skin, and superficial lesions due to lack of support for cutaneous blood vessels. Alterations in the immune responsiveness of the skin lead to a decreased response to surface inflammation (Balin & Allen, 1986).

Gastrointestinal System

Normal age-related changes in the gastrointestinal system are difficult to identify. Diminished functional capacity may be associated with normal aging; however, decreased functioning is more often due to disease states. Some age-related changes include mucosal changes, decreased blood flow to the organs, and changes in organ size and motility. Changes in the stomach with aging reflect atrophy of the gastric mucosa and a decreased production of hydrochloric acid. Alteration in surface area and function of the small intestine is thought to decrease absorption of certain essential nutrients, including vitamin D and calcium. Diminished motility of the colon and compromised blood flow to the large intestine characterize changes in the large intestine with age. Data do not support thinking that constipation is more common in older people despite changes in intestinal function. Rather, constipation in older adults may be due to drug therapy, inadequate hydration, or lack of dietary fiber (Singleton, 1990). Decreases in organ size and weight have been noted in the pancreas and liver with age. Fibrotic changes have been noted in pancreatic blood vessels with distention of the pancreatic ducts. Hepatic function is compromised, notably synthesis of cholesterol and total bile acid.

Genitourinary System

Many care providers and older patients view incontinence as a normal part of growing older (Branch, Walker, Wetle, DuBeau, & Resnick, 1994). However, incontinence may have serious negative consequences on the emotional and social well-being of older people (Urinary Incontinence Guideline Panel, 1992). Urinary incontinence poses a major problem for many elderly and plays a role in the development of rashes, pressure ulcers, urinary tract infections, and falls (Resnick & Ouslander, 1990; Urinary Incontinence Guideline Panel, 1992). Incontinence can limit daily activities and contribute to depression and anxiety. One reason for the increased prevalence of incontinence among older people may be associated chronic illnesses and functional impairments that become more common with age, rather than age itself (Resnick, 1995).

Anatomical and physiological changes occur in the genitourinary system with advanced age. Anatomical and physiological changes include loss of nephrons, progressive decrease in renal mass, and a decrease in the number of glomeruli. Sclerotic changes in renal blood vessels, particularly in hypertensive elderly people, lead to diminished renal blood flow and decreased creatinine clearance. Decreases in renal blood flow and glomerular filtration rate have been noted in response to age-related changes in cardiac output, renal mass, and decreased renal filtering surface. Creatinine clearance also decreases with age (Fillit & Rowe, 1992). A decline in endocrine functions of the kidney may be associated with a decrease in calcium absorption and anemia.

Bladder changes in older people include replacement of the smooth muscle and elastic tissue with fibrous connective tissue as well as a progressive weakening of bladder muscles and incomplete emptying. Bladder capacity is decreased in older people, with an associated increase in frequency of urination. Bladder contractility and the ability to postpone voiding appear to decline in both genders, whereas urethral length and closure pressure probably decline with age in women (Resnick, Elbadaw, & Yalla, 1995). The prostate enlarges in most men and appears to cause urodynamic obstruction in approximately 50% of elderly men (Resnick et al., 1995).

Musculoskeletal System

Normal age changes in the skeletal system of older people are often difficult to distinguish from the pathology of disease (Meier, 1997). Changes of the musculoskeletal system often are associated with diminished stature, a redistribution of lean body mass and subcutaneous fat, changes in bone density, muscle atrophy, diminished strength, and alterations in posture and mobility.

Musculoskeletal system changes with aging include a progressive decrease in stature, particularly among older women. This decrease is attributed to compression of the spinal column, narrowing of the intervertebral discs and loss of height of spinal vertebrae (Evans & Rosenberg, 1991; Matteson,

1997). The structure of the aging musculoskeletal system also is affected by changes in lean and fat mass distribution. As individuals age, the amount of lean body mass decreases, and subcutaneous fat increases and is redistributed. There is fat loss from the face and extremities and fat gain in abdomen and hips (Evans & Rosenberg, 1991). There is loss of skeletal calcium that accompanies normal aging. Following skeletal maturity, bone absorption begins to exceed bone formation. Age-related changes include reductions in gonadal hormone status, calcium intake, vitamin D status, physical activity, and other endocrine influences that negatively affect bone mass and metabolism (Meier, 1997). The progressive bone loss results in a loss of bone strength, estimated at 5% to 12% per decade from age 20 through 90, due primarily to a loss of bone mineral content (McArdle, Katch, & Katch, 1991).

Beginning at approximately age 40 to 50, a 10% to 20% decrease in muscle strength is expected, with a 30% to 40% decrease by age 70 to 80 (Collier & Arend, 1996). Muscle wasting is noted with increasing age due to a decrease in the number of muscle fibers. Regeneration of muscle tissue slows with age, and atrophied muscle tissue is replaced with fibrous tissue. The slower movement seen in aging individuals results from a prolongation of contraction time, latency period, and relaxation period of motor units in the muscle tissue (Stelmach, Populin, & Muller, 1990). There is a decrease in the size and number of type II muscle fibers, resulting in a reduction of isometric strength (Collier & Arend, 1996; Roos, Rice, & Vandervoort, 1997). Endurance does not appear to decline, as type I muscle fibers do not appear to atrophy with age (Frontera, Hughes, Lutz, & Evans, 1991; Rogers & Evans, 1993).

Alterations of posture and voluntary movement can be indicators of the health and biologic age of an individual. Age-associated limitations may affect quality of life by restricting mobility (Nutt, 1997). Voluntary movement slows with increasing age as a result of changes in the musculoskeletal and nervous systems. Postural changes may impair physical stability during movement and increase the risk for injury. Increased muscle rigidity and joint limitations also may impair movement. Age-related changes have been noted to occur in structural components of the joints, with decreases in function beginning after age 20 and accelerating after age 60 (Vandervoort et al., 1992).

Cardiovascular System

The changes with aging in the cardiovascular system include both structural and physiological changes, resulting in decreased cardiac reserve (Wenger, 1997). This decrease in reserve is not usually pronounced in the healthy elderly. However, aging effects may be observed when engaging in aerobic exercise, which challenges aerobic capacity and maximum heart rate. The overall size of the heart does not increase with aging, but there is a small increase in the left ventricular wall and ventricular septum (Wenger, 1997; Wenger, O'Rourke, & Marcus, 1988). The thickness of the left ventricular wall, ventricular septum, and overall weight of the heart increases with age, as do fat, collagen, and elastin, contributing to increased stiffness and decreased contractility.

The cardiac valves thicken and stiffen, and there is reduced diastolic compliance and filling (Kitzman & Edwards, 1990). Increased stiffness of the mitral and aortic valves may reflect accumulation of lipid, degeneration of collagen, and calcification of the valve fibrosa. These changes result in a decrease in maximum heart rate and maximal aerobic capacity (Wenger, 1997). Late diastolic filling increases with age due to decreased left ventricular compliance, decreased mitral valve competence, and prolonged relaxation. This results in decreased cardiac stroke volume and cardiac output (Wenger, 1997). Sympathetic tone is increased with age, resulting in supine resting cardiac output and stroke volume decreases. Upright cardiac reserve does not decrease (Wei & Gersh, 1987).

The conduction system in the aging heart also demonstrates changes. The number of pacemaker cells decreases significantly with age. There is loss of sinoatrial node cells; internodal tracts have an increase in fibrous tissue and fat, and calcification of the valves and conduction system occurs (Wenger, 1997).

Changes in the peripheral vascular system underlie the changes in blood pressure that accompany aging (Rowe & Lipsitz, 1988). There are changes in the vascular smooth muscle, including aortic and large artery thickness and vascular stiffness, which contribute to left ventricular ejection impedance and increased systolic pressure (Wenger, 1997).

Pulmonary System

There are both structural and functional changes in the elderly individual that predispose to alterations in respiratory function over time. These changes result in an increase in the work of breathing, decrease in reserve capacity, reduction in flow rates, and decrease in cough effectiveness in older people (McClaran, Babcock, Pegelow, Reddan, & Dempsey, 1995). There is a loss of pulmonary reserve with aging. Increased stiffness of the chest wall due to osteoporosis of the ribs and vertebrae, calcification of the costal cartilages, and diminished muscle strength contribute to reduced maximal inspiratory and expiratory force (Johnson & Dempsey, 1991).

The major effect of the aging process on the pulmonary system is the reduced quality of gas exchange in the lungs so that less oxygen reaches the blood (Webster & Cain, 1997). There are progressive losses of lung elastic recoil, and the alveoli enlarge and become thinner, reducing surface area for gas exchange (Johnson & Dempsey, 1991). Total lung capacity remains essentially constant with age. The residual volume may increase with age, due to airway collapse at higher lung volumes secondary to loss of elastic recoil (McClaran et al., 1995).

Neurological System

Researchers and clinicians have focused their efforts on understanding the effects of physiological aging on cognitive, emotional, and behavioral functioning (Koltai & Chelune, 1996). Critical to these efforts has been the identification of reliable methods to discern those cognitive effects that occur during normal aging from degenerative dementing diseases (Smith, Malec, & Ivnik, 1992). Changes in the neurological system are manifested in functional changes for the elderly individual. The generalized slowing and wasting of the nervous system accompanying aging affects several functional areas. Functional changes that occur with aging include a slowing of reaction time (Mucignat, Castiello, Umilta, & Tradard, 1991), loss of sensory cues, decline in function of muscle stretch receptors, and associated loss of muscle mass (Maki, Holliday, & Topper, 1994; Pyykko, Jantti, & Aalto, 1990; Stelmach et al., 1990). There are decreases in visual acuity and accommodation, as well as often-marked changes in auditory function.

Structural changes that occur with normal aging include loss of neurons, slowed synaptic transmissions, and loss of peripheral nerve function. Changes in prefrontal and subcortical brain regions are thought to be part of the normal aging process that leads to many of the declines in cognitive functioning in older people (Gur, Gur, Obrist, Skolnick, & Reivich, 1987). With advancing age, there is thought to be a slowing in central nervous system processing (Salthouse, 1991), which reduces cognitive speed and negatively affects cognitive function. The speed and potential to process auditory and visual information, particularly novel information, is diminished in older people (Kausler, Wiley, & Lieberwitz, 1992). A change in memory is probably the most frequent concern of older people (Dobbs & Rule, 1989). Empirical findings have shown that for the most part, short-term memory is well preserved into old age (Albert, 1994). However, age-related effects are evident on tasks that require recall and recognition of verbal and visual materials (Koltai & Chelune, 1996). It is felt that in the healthy elderly, age-associated memory impairment reflects a nondementing aging process. This is defined as the absence of medical conditions that could contribute to memory impairment, a memory test performance at least one standard deviation below the mean of young adults, and subjective memory complaints.

Endocrine System

Age-related changes in the endocrine system affect both the reception and the production of hormones. Alterations have been noted in the structure and function of the pituitary and thyroid glands, adrenal cortex, gonads, parathyroid glands, and pancreas. Additional changes that occur in the older man include decrease in testicular volume and spermatogenesis. Testosterone secretion declines, and there is an increase in estrogen-to-testosterone ratio. Women experience menopause and decreased serum estrogen production. Endocrine changes that occur with aging affect metabolic processes. In women, cessation of menses accompanies reduced estrogen production and decreased follicular sensitivity to gonadotropins. Changes in pancreatic function result in a decreased glucose tolerance and a corresponding decline in insulin secretion.

In summary, a wide variation in physical and physiological changes accompany aging. The degree to which these changes affect the elderly individual's quality of life may depend on the degree to which the individual responds to the changes. Health promotion efforts can reduce the unfavorable individual responses to the changes of aging; prevention efforts can distinguish between those changes that are normal and gradual and those that become pathological and lead to disease.

FUNCTIONAL ASSESSMENT

A major defining characteristic of good health for older people is functional ability or functional status. The ability to function independently is a primary interest of older persons and should be a primary focus of health care. Although not all older persons are ill and disabled, a significant minority reports some activity limitation due to chronic disease or impairment (Kaplan, 1997). Data indicate that approximately 42% of women and 66% men over the age of 75 years are unable to perform heavy household work. Forty-two percent of women over 75 years cannot stand for more than 15 minutes, 20% are unable to climb stairs, and 33% cannot lift a weight of more than 10 pounds (Branch, Katz, Kneipman, & Papsidero, 1984). Similarly, the number of days in which an older person is required to limit usual activities due to illness or injury is reported to be approximately 35 days per year, as compared with 14 days for persons 25 to 44 years of age. Women 65 and older report more restricted activity days than their male counterparts.

Although the presence of a single chronic disease may lead to disability, the impact of multiple chronic conditions, or *comorbidities,* on disability status is considerable. High rates of comorbidity have been reported for women, with prevalence rates rising from 45% for women 60 to 69 years of age to 70% for women 80 and over.

Thorough and appropriate assessment of the elderly individual is critical to the development of intervention strategies directed toward risk reduction and health promotion. Physical, social, and mental factors are intertwined in the assessment of older individuals (Kane, 1990). Comprehensive geriatric assessment (CGA), the "new technology" of geriatrics, is a multidisciplinary, multidimensional diagnostic process that assesses an individual's functional and psychosocial capabilities and medical problems to develop an overall treatment plan (Rubenstein, Wieland, & Bernabei, 1995). The CGA is comprehensive: It emphasizes quality of life and functional status and uses standardized measurement instruments. The goal of the CGA is to achieve more comprehensive diagnoses, detect and evaluate distinct problems, and integrate them into long-term planning. The basic components of the CGA include evaluation of medical problems, psychological status, functional status, social support network, economic needs, and the living environment (Rubenstein et al., 1995). A major component in the CGA is the evaluation of the elderly individual's functional status. This assessment provides information to the health care team on the individual's ability to live in the community.

Comprehensive functional assessment includes both the nature and extent of functional ability. Physical health can be measured by combinations of diagnoses, symptoms, disabilities, and self-reports and should include screening for vision, hearing, or dental problems. Functional assessment is generally classified into two areas: activities of daily living and instrumental activities. Daily living activities are linked to self-care and independent living assessments. Most fundamental activities include bathing, dressing, transferring, continence, and eating. Instrumental activities include cooking, cleaning, laundry, preparing meals, driving, managing money, and taking medications. The assessment of mental and emotional stability is assessed using measures of depression differentiating saddened mood states from sustained and severe depression. Examining social contacts, relationships, social roles, resources, and activities assesses social functioning. Frequency of social contacts may be counted, but the satisfaction of the contacts, critical to functional status, is very subjective. Assessment of mental functioning is the interaction of cognitive and affective status. Cognition includes memory, perception, judgment, calculation, and social integrity (Kane, 1990).

Numerous standardized measures are available to assess functional status. Among these are the Katz Index of Activities of Daily Living (Katz, Ford, Moskowitz, Jackson, & Jaffe, 1963), the Barthel Index (Mahoney & Barthel, 1965), the Rapid Disability Rating Scale (Linn & Linn, 1982), and the Physical Performance Test (Reuben & Siu, 1990).

The purposes of standardized measures are to record the individual's functional assessment and gauge limitations of capability and performance. Standardized measures are used to monitor changes over time and estimate the efficacy of interventions. Standardized measures are important in that they may provide more precise, unbiased, and reproducible assessments. For example, the clinical judgment of impairment is not consistently related to the measurement of impairment, nor can clinical judgment discover moderate impairment (Pinholt et al., 1987).

Several issues surround the use of standard assessment instruments. A major issue is the selection of the "norms" against which an instrument is standardized. This is an important issue, because pathologic findings are assessed against norms to ascertain their normal distribution. However, caution must be made concerning these norms, as functional deviations that are labeled "impairments" may not actually be impairments but may be common in the population (Kane, 1990). The threshold of the measuring instrument is important; the threshold is the definition below which the observed event becomes a problem (Kane, 1990). As with any measurement, the cultural basis of the instrument and the recipient must be considered, as differences may be based on ethnicity and social class. Reliability and validity are critical elements to assess in any instrument that assesses functional status. Reliability is the extent to which findings are repeatable, and validity, the extent to which the instrument measures what it is intended to measure. Last, the instrument's use in a practical sense must be considered. For example, does the instrument differentiate between capability and performance—that is, can it measure the extent to which an individual can bathe himself or herself versus the extent to which they do bathe themselves (Kane, 1990)? Capability can be demonstrated through self-report or demonstration. The time and place of measurement is an important consideration; familiar surroundings are likely to provide more accurate descriptions than unfamiliar settings, such as a hospital.

In summary, the assessment of the older individual's functional ability is one important way to determine the health promotion needs and requirements for services (Matteson, 1997). Health promotion efforts are primarily directed toward the prevention of lifestyle-related declines in capabilities. Secondary prevention efforts are targeted toward the reduction of the sequelae of disease-related declines in function.

CHAPTER 2

Health Risk in Older People

A mong the most compelling reasons to encourage health promotion efforts in older people relate to the use of health care services. Capitation through managed care and major incentives to reduce health care use hallmark the direction and success of health promotion and disease prevention strategies to reduce utilization demands by older people (Fries, Bloch, Harrington, Richardson, & Beck, 1993; Fries, Koop, et al., 1993). Many of the chronic disabilities of older people are related to unfavorable lifestyles, and health promotion efforts can reduce the unfavorable sequelae of aging (U.S. Department of Health and Human Services [USDHHS], 1991). The health risks and opportunities for health promotion targets the areas of cigarette smoking, sedentary lifestyle, nutritional risk, and stressors are discussed in this chapter.

CIGARETTE SMOKING

Cigarette smoking remains the leading preventable cause of morbidity and premature mortality in the United States. More than 4,000 substances have been identified in cigarette smoke, many of which are toxic, mutagenic, carcinogenic, and pharmacologically active. Smoking causes an increase in the aging process of the lung, decreased pulmonary function, and an increase in morbidity and mortality in older people. Older individuals who continue to smoke are also at greater risk for cerebral and cardiovascular complications, osteoporosis, loss of mobility, and reduced physical function.

A number of studies have indicated an increased risk of mortality associated with smoking in aged populations (Kaplan, Seeman, Cohen, Knudsen, &
Guralnik, 1987; LaCroix et al., 1991; Schoenfeld, Malmrose, Blazer, Gold,
& Seeman, 1994). Cigarette smoking lowers the age of initial myocardial
infarction (MI) more for women than for men (Hansen, Andersen, & Von
Eyben, 1993) and imparts a threefold greater risk of MI in women, including
premenopausal women compared with men (Willett et al., 1987). In an examination of mortality risk as a function of smoking history, Kaplan et al.
(1987) found that those individuals who continued to smoke over a 9-year
study period had a 76% increased risk of mortality compared with those
who had never smoked. In contrast, those who quit smoking during the study
period had a 33% increased risk. Smoking cessation following coronary
artery bypass surgery in patients in the Coronary Artery Surgery Study registry improved survival in both men and women, with the benefit persisting
into older age (Hermanson, Omenn, Kronmal, & Gersh, 1988).

In addition to the increased risk for mortality, smoking also may have a
significant impact on morbidity levels and functional status in older age.
Data indicate that nonsmokers and former smokers have higher levels of
physical function compared with continuing smokers (Kaplan, 1997). In a
19-year follow-up of participants in the Alameda County Study, those who
were smokers at study initiation were twice as likely to have experienced
a reduction in physical function, including activities of daily living, compared with those who had never smoked (Guralnik & Kaplan, 1989). In a
4-year longitudinal study examining the relation between smoking and
mobility among functional adults, LaCroix, Guralnik, Berkman, Wallace,
and Satterfield (1993) found that those who were current smokers at baseline had the highest rate of loss of mobility. In a 6-year study examining
changes in physical function related to smoking status, Kaplan, Strawbridge,
Camacho, and Cohen (1993) found that physical function was related to smoking status, with current smokers showing greater declines in functioning than
did those who were former smokers and those who had never smoked.

Cigarette smoking has been identified as an independent and significant
risk factor for the development of coronary heart disease (CHD). In almost all
studies, a dose-response gradient has been documented between the number
of cigarettes smoked daily and the incidence of CHD. Smoking confers a twofold to sixfold increased risk of both CHD and nonfatal MI compared to never
smoking (LaCroix et al., 1993). In almost all studies, a dose-response gradient has been documented between the number of cigarettes smoked daily
and the incidence of CHD. Those who quit smoking have lower death rates
than do people who continue to smoke. In addition, cigarette smoking acts

synergistically with other risk factors to increase greatly the risk for CHD in older people. Epidemiological studies have documented a strong risk association between cigarette smoking and cardiovascular outcomes, including CHD, peripheral vascular disease, stroke, and increased mortality (Kannel & Higgins, 1990).

Smoking-induced transient cardiovascular responses in healthy people include an increased heart rate and blood pressure, cardiac stroke volume and output, and decreased coronary blood flow. Concentrations of free fatty acids, glycerol, and lactate are increased. Carbon monoxide from cigarette smoke also produces cardiovascular effects, including hypoxia of the intima and an increase in endothelial permeability. Increased platelet aggregation, increased platelet adhesiveness, shortened platelet survival, decreased clotting times, and an increased hematocrit have been recorded in smokers (Muller, Abela, Nesto, & Tofler, 1994). In animal studies, cardiac automaticity has been shown to increase, and the threshold for ventricular fibrillation is lowered. These effects may account for the increased risk of sudden death observed in cigarette smokers. Smoking cessation confers benefits irrespective of gender, age, or other comorbidities. Smoking status should be assessed in all patients in the primary care and community setting and smoking cessation encouraged among all elderly individuals who smoke.

PHYSICAL INACTIVITY

Because older individuals experience a progressive decline in many physiologic functions, including muscular strength and cardiovascular capacity, physical activity can provide many of the benefits of exercise for a substantial number of older adults. Physical activity can be considered an important component of overall health promotion for older people.

Although it is assumed that physical illness leads to functional limitations, the causal relation may be the other way around. Bortz (1996) coined the term *disuse syndrome,* a set of six conditions commonly seen in older people derived from lack of body vigor due to disuse. The disuse syndrome includes cardiovascular vulnerability, musculoskeletal fragility, immunologic susceptibility, obesity, depression, and premature aging. Low functional aerobic capacity and reduced voluntary physical activity are associated with all cause-specific mortality rates from chronic disease such as CHD, diabetes, and cancer (Blair et al., 1989).

Blair et al. (1989) studied 13,000 men and women, ranked into quintiles according to fitness, for an average of 8 years. Those who were the most fit survived longest. The greatest differential in survival was between those who reported no physical activity and those who reported doing a little. In other words, the most important step was the first one. The second major finding from Blair et al.'s (1989) study was that the older we become, the more important fitness is to survival. By age 70, there is a sevenfold difference in survival between those who are least fit and those who are most fit; this advantage is only marginal in younger adults.

Older adults with a sedentary lifestyle when compared to older adults with an active lifestyle have a 1.53% increase in risk of dying (Kannel, 1997; Sherman, D'Agostino, Cobb, & Kannel, 1994). Some of the physical limitations older people experience are a direct result of the natural process of aging, such as genetic or hormonal effects. However, age-related decline in part can be attributed to the effects of an adverse lifestyle. The physical activity an individual has had throughout his or her lifetime contributes to health outcomes. In a retrospective study comparing physically active and inactive elderly women, the cumulative difference between physically active and sedentary women was apparent by age 25 and persisted through life (Voorrips, Lemmink, Van Heuvelen, Bult, & Van Staveren, 1993).

Reports from cardiac exercise programs reveal that, on average, half of the patients who start a program never finish. In studies of exercise adherence, drop-out rates range from 20% to 60%, with the lowest attrition occurring during the first 3 months of a program. Fifty percent of exercise dropout occurs between 6 and 12 months in both supervised and unsupervised exercise programs (Dishman, 1990).

Falls

One of the most deleterious outcomes of reduced muscle strength, bone strength, and joint mobility is the heightened susceptibility of older individuals, particularly women, to falls and to serious consequences resulting from falls (Lord & Castell, 1994a, 1994b; Lord, Caplan, & Ward, 1993). Community survey estimates of the prevalence of falling range from 32% (Tinetti, Speechley, & Ginter, 1988) to 42% (Downton & Andrews, 1990).

Foremost of all medical conditions experienced by the older person is both the risk of and actual occurrence of a fall. The experience of a fall can lead to a cycle in which one fall leads the individual to become fearful of more falls, and, as a result, to walk less securely and confidently. This loss of a sense of security can serve to increase the risk that older persons will lose their balance and make them more likely to fall in the future (Omenn et al., 1997).

It is estimated that each year there are more than 30 million falls (Hayes et al., 1996). The most severe consequence of a fall—hip fracture—results from only about 1% of falls, yet a hip fracture accounts for the majority of cost and disability associated with a fall (Hayes et al., 1996). In addition, disability can result from loss of confidence, fear of falling, and deteriorating function. Elderly women experience hip fracture resulting from falls more than do elderly men, and this may be attributed to less bone mineral density in women. Identification of the factors that contribute to the risk of falls is an important assessment skill for the clinician. In addition, because most falls are avoidable, efforts by the clinician to reduce safety and functional limitations, as well as to strengthen the older person's muscle strength, balance, and coordination, offer an important health promotion consideration for the vulnerable elderly.

There are a number of interacting age-related processes that operate to increase the older adult's likelihood of suffering from a disabling fall, including musculoskeletal changes and sensory losses (Woollacott, 1993) and an increased likelihood of tripping over obstacles (Chen, Ashton-Miller, Alexander, & Schultz, 1994). Those elderly who are most at risk of falling include people who suffer, in addition to bone loss, from visual impairment, neurological deficits, gait disturbance, loss of muscle strength and coordination, and health problems requiring certain medications (Lord & Castell, 1994a, 1994b; Lord et al., 1993; Maki, Holliday, & Topper, 1991).

Osteoporosis

Osteoporosis occurs as a result of both aging and menopause. A gradual decline in bone density occurs throughout middle age and is accelerated following menopause (Lindsay, 1993). Estrogen is an important determinant of bone loss, and inactivity augments the loss. Bone remodeling occurs in bone remodeling units. Osteoclasts appear on previously inactive bone surfaces and excavate a lacuna or resorption tunnel. Osteoblasts then replace the osteoclasts, refilling the resorption cavity. Bone loss is increased if this remodeling balance becomes upset (Turner, Riggs, & Spelsberg, 1994). Osteoblastic and osteoclastic activity in the bone tissue is altered by interleukins and is implicated in postmenopausal osteoporosis (Breder, Dinarello, & Saper, 1988). Sex steroids impact bone physiology in several ways: They maintain mineral homeostasis during reproduction, maintain bone balance, and, when diminished, predispose bone to loss and osteoporotic fractures (Turner et al., 1994).

Bone remodeling occurs as a result of ovarian insufficiency (estrogen deficiency; Lindsay, Bush, Grady, Speroff, & Lobo, 1996). The bone remodeling is hypothesized to result in a shift that favors bone resorption. In addition, remodeling increases the opportunity for trabecular penetration during resorption, that is, loss of the template upon which new bone is built and loss of bone tissue (Dempster & Lindsay, 1993). With diminished estrogen, there is an increase in the activation of new bone remodeling units, resulting in remodeling imbalance. Osteoclasts construct deeper resorption spaces, and there is impairment of the ability of osteoblasts to refill them (Turner et al., 1994).

Estrogen maintains bone mass by supplying cancellous bone remodeling and maintaining the balance between osteoblastic and osteoclastic activity (Turner et al., 1994). It is hypothesized that the action of estrogen receptors on bone cells is direct, although this is unclear (Turner et al., 1994).

NUTRITIONAL RISK

Maintaining good nutrition is important for health promotion and disease prevention among older people. Dietary intake has been identified as an important component in the prevention and management of many chronic conditions, including CHD, diabetes mellitus, and hypertension. With advancing age, the risk of developing nutritional deficiencies increases due to age-related reductions in total food intake combined with the presence of debilitating disease. The presence of malnutrition increases functional dependency, morbidity, mortality, and the use of health care resources. Similarly, nutritional intake greater than body requirements has made obesity among older people a primary public health problem in the United States.

Overnutrition

Obesity is a major health problem in the United States, particularly among older people. Increases in body weight resulting in obesity represent an important risk factor for chronic disease in older people. Body fat distribution, being overweight, and obesity are independent predictors of cardiovascular disease in some populations (McGinnis & Ballard-Barbash, 1991). Among 5,209 men and women of the original Framingham cohort, obesity was a significant independent predictor of cardiovascular disease, particularly among women (Hubert, Feinleib, McNamara, & Castelli, 1983). Increases in body weight have been associated with cardiovascular risk factors, including elevated blood pressure, increased serum cholesterol and triglyceride levels, and increased blood glucose levels. Obesity is associated with an atherogenic lipoprotein profile (National Research Council, 1989). Obesity has been negatively related to high-density lipoprotein cholesterol (HDL-C), including HDL_2 and HDL_3, and positively correlated with plasma total cholesterol, low-density lipoprotein cholesterol (LDL-C), and triglyceride levels (Grundy, 1994; Kris-Etherton, 1990). Kannel (1990), reporting Framingham data, estimated that, in women, for each percent increase in relative weight, there was predicted a 0.6 mg/dl increase in serum cholesterol. Dattilo and Kris-Etherton (1992) reported that blood lipid profiles demonstrate improvement with weight loss alone.

Data substantiate the importance of obesity as an independent contributor to the development of CHD (Leiter et al., 1994; Manson et al., 1990). Recent studies also emphasize the importance of body fat distribution in conferring risk for developing CHD (Bjorntorp, 1990, 1992). Patterns of increased abdominal or truncal obesity have been associated with hypertension, hyperlipidemia, insulin resistance, very low density lipoprotein cholesterol (VLDL-C) and triglycerides, and low concentrations of HDL-C, all of which increase cardiovascular risk (Reaven, 1993). Furthermore, abdominal obesity has been directly associated with cardiovascular morbidity and mortality (Anderson & Kannel, 1992). Greater waist-to-hip ratios are independently associated with increased prevalence of hypertension, diabetes mellitus, stroke, and postload serum glucose concentration (Folsom et al., 1991).

Undernutrition

Some data have indicated that being underweight is associated with as high a mortality rate as moderate obesity, particularly in those over 60 years of age. Data from the Elderly Nutrition Program of the Older Americans Act showed that 67% to 88% of participants were at nutritional risk (Kennedy, Ohls, Carlson, & Fleming, 1995). According to data presented in the Position Statement of the American Dietetic Association, 8% to 16% of older adults do not have regular access to a nutritionally adequate, culturally compatible diet (Kennedy et al., 1995). Clinically, a number of important questions must be addressed in the nutritional assessment. Increased risk of malnutrition usually can be identified from the history and physical examination. Factors leading to malnutrition can be categorized into disorders resulting in anorexia, inadequate or inappropriate nutrient intake, and social or economic isolation. Approximately 20% of older adults are poor, with older women making up a higher percentage compared with older men. Those who live alone or with nonfamily members, who represent a minority group, have lower levels of education, or who are unable to work are more likely to be poor (Census Bureau, 1990).

STRESSORS AMONG VULNERABLE
INDIVIDUALS AND GROUPS

Individual health behaviors, lifestyle practices, environmental and psycho-social stresses, and availability of health care resources all contribute to health promotion behaviors among the vulnerable elderly. Vulnerability in health matters, including health prevention and health promotion, is affected by factors that have isolated or marginalized groups from resources, services, and educational and occupational advantages. The vulnerable elderly include women and individuals from diverse ethnic and racial backgrounds. The minority-group elderly population is growing faster than that of whites and will continue to do so. It is estimated that by 2015, 15% of the elderly popula-tion will be nonwhite, and that by 2025, 20% will be nonwhite (Agnee, 1986). In the United States, many subgroups of the population have considerably worse health than the population as a whole and therefore deserve priority for public health promotion efforts. Impaired health and elevated health risks in numerous respects have been documented in African Americans, Hispanics/ Latinos, American Indians, Alaskan Natives, Pacific Islanders, and Asian Americans, as well as among immigrant groups, rural dwellers, and the poor.

Sociocultural Barriers to Health Promotion Efforts

Sociocultural and socioeconomic status (SES) has a significant impact on the health of minority groups (Johnson et al., 1995). Examinations of health issues in cultural and ethnic groups emphasize the within-group diversity that exists among various cultures, thus making cultural generalizations difficult (Flack et al., 1995). Diversity within and across ethnic groups has been attrib-uted to differences in country of origin, culture, degree of acculturation, and SES (Nickens, 1995). The dramatic differences in the four recognized minor-ity groups serve to alert the health care provider to differences in risk assess-ment and interventions among cultural and ethnic groups.

Cultural barriers are instrumental in decisions to use or not use the formal medical system, for both health screening and health promotion efforts. Ac-cess to medical care, acceptance of therapeutic interventions, and health edu-cation efforts depend on many factors, including cultural values. For exam-ple, among African Americans, discomfort and distrust of the health care system and providers may hamper health promotion efforts (Flack et al., 1995). Social and political power is diminished in vulnerable groups, and this diminution of power is linked with poor health outcomes (LaVeist, 1992).

In many situations, language and social barriers hallmark isolation from mainstream health services (Hopper, 1993). Acculturation of immigrant Americans, regardless of their ethnic affiliation, produces significant stresses. Adaptation to the host culture's economic and social system and disruption of existing social support networks have been related to poor health (Kaplan & Marks, 1990).

Racial differences such as skin color among ethnic groups affects health promotion efforts as a cultural barrier, in that skin color frequently acts as a barrier to desirable resources (Johnson et al., 1995). Investigators have found a relation between gender, racial discrimination, and adverse health consequences. Racism is particularly apparent in the lack of cultural sensitivity to groups who participate in nontraditional healing practices (Johnson et al., 1995).

Elderly minority women are among the most vulnerable in the aged population. Some factors that contribute to this group's vulnerability include limited income, poor education, substandard housing, malnutrition, and diminished initial health status (Hopper, 1993).

Socioeconomic Barriers to Health Promotion Efforts

Patterns of aging and the quality of life of old people are closely related to the economic and social health of society at large. Although most older persons are not poor, the range of economic differences among older people is very wide. The poverty rate for individuals 65 years and older dropped from 24.6% in 1970 to 12.2% in 1993 (Census Bureau, 1990). These data are misleading, however, because the threshold for poverty for older adults is lower; thus, the true prevalence of poverty may be biased (Institute of Medicine, 1993). About as many older men have very high incomes as do the number who live in poverty (i.e., fewer than 10%; Census Bureau, 1990). The distribution is different for women, of whom a larger proportion (15%) have incomes under the poverty level.

Elderly women enter old age poorer than elderly men (Meyer, 1990). This incidence of poverty is linked to their likelihood of being widowed or divorced. The majority of women over 65 are widowed and have been in the labor force only intermittently; as a consequence, they have little or no social security or pension benefits of their own. Along with entering old age poorer than men, older women, as a consequence of widowhood, health care expenses, and pension inequities, experience increasing poverty as they age (Minkler & Stone, 1985). Very old widowed women and single women are particularly disadvantaged: From 23% to 28% have incomes below the poverty level. Thus, the term "feminization of poverty" has come to characterize the older woman (Hopper, 1993).

Minority elderly, especially African Americans, are very disadvantaged. Thirty-three percent of African Americans live below the poverty level. Hispanics have the lowest socioeconomic attainment of all ethnic groups in the United States; unemployment is 40% to 60% higher than their white counterparts (Census Bureau, 1990). Mexican Americans are 2.5 times more likely to live below the poverty level than their white counterparts (Census Bureau, 1990). American Indians, compared to non-Indians, are two to three times more likely to live in poverty (Johnson et al., 1995).

For many minorities in the United States, low SES exerts a powerful negative influence on health resources and health status. Hispanics are more likely than whites or African Americans to have no health insurance, thus creating barriers for health screening and promotion efforts (Johnson et al., 1995). Low income and education is disparately prevalent among African American and Hispanic women because the prevalence of poverty is three times that of whites (Census Bureau, 1990).

Across these vulnerable groups, the social and economic disadvantages that have accumulated throughout their lives are accentuated in old age. A lifetime exposure to low or inadequate economic conditions is associated with health risk. For example, exposure to occupational hazards and carcinogens may be higher for individuals with poor job conditions and limited education (Aday, 1993; Johnson et al., 1995). Lack of childhood health care may set the stage for acute and chronic illness processes that may be difficult to treat (Johnson et al., 1995).

The use of preventive services by older people is strongly influenced by poverty. Poverty may reduce the likelihood of the use of preventive services, as medical and preventive services are less likely to be located in poor neighborhoods. The lack of economic and social resources constrains individuals who live in areas with a high population of households in poverty, preventing them from using services and interventions targeted at risk reduction and health promotion. Concern for food, shelter, and clothing characterizes the priorities for elderly living in poverty. Health prevention and health promotion efforts do not take precedence over survival needs. This makes the receipt of health care discontinuous and focused on alleviation of medical symptoms rather than on prevention.

Even when health care services are available, low SES individuals tend to use preventive health services less than do individuals with higher SES (Katz & Hofer, 1994). For example, low-income women, particularly ethnic minority women, are less likely to obtain screening mammograms than are other groups of women (Hedegaard, Davidson, & Wright, 1996). Racial and ethnic variations are the strongest predictors of breast cancer screening practices. Ethnic minority women are less likely to conduct clinical and self-breast exams and report less frequent mammography use (Pearlman, Rakowski, Ehrich, & Clark, 1996). When entire neighborhoods are poor, individuals are less likely to know about or be encouraged by communities to use preventive services (Breen & Figueroa, 1996). Women living in poverty engage in fewer breast and cervical cancer screening practices, and living in an impoverished neighborhood consistently predicts the occurrence of invasive cancer (Breen & Figueroa, 1996).

African American Elderly. The most salient disparity in minority health is between African Americans and white Americans. African Americans have a life expectancy 5 to 7 years less than that of their white counterparts (National Center for Health Statistics, 1997). The overall life expectancy for African Americans in 1991 was an average of 69.3 years; in white Americans, the average age expectancy was 76.3 years (National Center for Health Statistics, 1997). The leading cause of death among African Americans is cardiovascular disease, followed by cancer, with the ratio of death for those diseases between African Americans and white Americans being 6 to 1 and 2 to 1, respectively (Nickens, 1995). In addition, racial differences continue to exist in the equality of health care provided to African Americans.

The health profile of African Americans is more detrimental than that of their white counterparts (Kumanyika & Golden, 1991; Myers, Kagawa-Singer, Kumanyika, Lex, & Markides, 1995). This health profile is composed of health risk behaviors and contributes to the disproportionate mortality and morbidity of African Americans (Kumanyika, 1993). Although the incidence of breast cancer among African American women is lower than that among white women, their survival is poorer. This is attributed to the more advanced stage of the disease when it is diagnosed (Eley et al., 1994). Among African American women, the prognosis for several gynecologic cancers is poorer, and there is an increased mortality and decreased 5-year survival as compared to whites (Roach et al., 1997). Older African American women have a higher prevalence of hypertension, diabetes, and obesity than do African American men and individuals from other racial and ethnic origins (Farrell, Kohl, & Rogers, 1987). In addition, African American women report poorer functional status and quality of life than do other groups (Farrell et al., 1987).

Dietary fat intake in African Americans is higher than in the average white American (Kumanyika, 1990, 1993; Kumanyika, Morssink, & Agurs, 1992).

Sixty percent of 45- to 74-year-old African American women are over-weight; the prevalence of those overweight in African American men between the ages of 35 and 54 is 40% (Myers et al., 1995). Fewer African American men than white men exercise, and there is a decline in physical activity after age 64. At all age groups, African American women are less inclined to exercise than their white counterparts (Schoenborn & Marano, 1988). In African Americans, a major risk factor that contributes to chronic illness and hampers health promotion efforts is the high rate of smoking (Johnson et al., 1995). Among African American women, examinations of health seeking behavior show that illness is first treated at home, and individuals seek health care less frequently and delay longer than their white counterparts (Gibbs, 1988). The reluctance that African American individuals demonstrate in preventive health seeking behavior has been attributed to fear and distrust of health care providers (Myers et al., 1995).

Hispanic/Latino Elderly. In 1990, non-Hispanic whites made up about 75% of the population of the United States. It is projected that, by the year 2050, the United States will be about one half minority (Census Bureau, 1990). Hispanics represent more than 9% of the United States population, with more than 22.3 million individuals in the continental United States (Census Bureau, 1990). Mexican Americans constitute the largest subgroup and are distributed primarily in the Southwest. Puerto Ricans follow in size, primarily living on the East Coast, with Cubans the third-largest Hispanic subgroup, living primarily in Florida (Census Bureau, 1990).

Among the morbidity and mortality data that is salient to the aging Hispanic population is the high prevalence of non-insulin-dependent diabetes mellitis (NIDDM). This chronic illness is two to three times higher in Hispanics than in non-Hispanic whites (National Center for Health Statistics, 1997). Puerto Ricans have a poorer health status than do other Hispanic groups. For Puerto Ricans, the death rate from cardiovascular disease is disproportionately higher than for other Hispanic groups (National Center for Health Statistics, 1997). Compared with other Americans, Hispanic Americans are at a higher risk for other diseases. For example, Hispanics are disproportionately afflicted with AIDS, tuberculosis, and unintentional injuries (USDHHS, 1991).

Hispanic Americans, compared to whites and African Americans, demonstrate a relatively low use of health services (USDHHS, 1991). Among Hispanic women, factors that contribute to less frequent use of health services, particularly those that involve gynecologic matters, include the influence of traditional gender roles, such as extreme modesty (Markides & Vernon, 1984).

Asians and Pacific Island Elderly. Asians and Pacific Islanders number 1.3 million in the United States, are the fastest growing ethnic group in this country, and demonstrate significant diversity in language, culture, and geographic distribution (Census Bureau, 1990). According to the Census Bureau, this heterogeneous group includes Asians (Japanese, Chinese, Koreans, and Filipinos) and Pacific Islanders (Hawaiians, Samoans, Togans, Guamanians, and Fijians).

Health knowledge about this diverse group is sparse and is confounded by inadequate data. What is known is that there is disproportionate use of health care services and that poverty and overcrowded living conditions are prevalent in high-density urban settings (Johnson et al., 1995). The Chinese have a tuberculosis rate four times higher than the national average, and preventive health care is not a priority for Asian immigrants (Johnson et al., 1995). Members of the Japanese, Chinese, and Filipino ethnic groups have lower death rates than do white Americans (Liu & Yu, 1985). However, adoption of the Western lifestyle and diet has increased the risk of diseases such as CHD, diabetes, and obesity (Fujimoto et al., 1987). For Asian American women, depression and suicide are significant health problems, particularly among the older Chinese and Japanese women (Hopper, 1993).

Health risk behaviors related to chronic illness are difficult to obtain in Asians and Pacific Islanders. There is a misconception that the low use of health care services among this group is equated with good health (Flack et al., 1995; Myers et al., 1995). Other than Koreans, who exercise at one third to one fifth the proportion of white Americans, no information is known about health promotion behavior in the larger cultural group of Asians-Pacific Islanders (Stavig, Igra, & Leonard, 1988). Smoking rates for acculturated Asians-Pacific Islanders are comparable, except for Southeast Asians, who have rates of 54% to 92% (Chen, Kuun, Guthrie, & Zaharlick, 1991).

Numerous barriers to access of preventive health care exist among Asian Americans. These include language barriers, economic issues, and cultural stigmas attributed to certain medical disorders (Hopper, 1993).

Native American Elderly. American Indians live in small, complex, and discrete populations, with more than 200 distinct tribes (Flack et al., 1995). Chronic illnesses such as cancer have relatively low impact on morbidity and mortality in this group, whereas NIDDM has a remarkably high prevalence (Flack et al., 1995). A Native American has 10 times the likelihood of developing NIDDM (USDHHS, 1991). In this group, heart disease, stroke, and cancer are the leading causes of death but are lower in prevalence than among all other ethnic groups (USDHHS, 1991). Compared with other older individuals, the American Indian in the United States lives in worse socioeconomic conditions, experiences functional decline faster, and becomes frail sooner (Cuellar, 1990). Obesity among Native Americans has a high prevalence and is coupled with a sedentary lifestyle among 40% to 65% of men and women in this group (Sugarman, Warren, Oge, & Helgerson, 1992).

CARDIOVASCULAR RISK IN OLDER PEOPLE

Atherosclerosis is a pathologic condition of the arteries clinically manifested as cardiovascular disease, the major cause of death in the industrialized world. Coronary artery disease and cerebrovascular disease, both of which are atherosclerotic diseases, cause more death, disability, and economic loss in the United States than any other disease (American Heart Association, 1998). The incidence of almost all cardiovascular diseases increases with advancing age, emphasizing the need for cardiovascular risk assessment and health promotion efforts in older people.

Several risk factors have been linked to the presence or acceleration of the atherosclerotic process in older people. Modifiable risk factors that affect the prognosis for a person with or at risk for cardiovascular disease include (a) lifestyle influences such as cigarette smoking, dietary patterns associated with obesity, and sedentary lifestyle; and (b) atherogenic personal traits, including hypertension, hyperlipidemia, diabetes mellitus, and psychosocial factors. Reduction or elimination of these risk factors also has been linked to a reduced death rate from cardiovascular disease and stroke and regression of atherosclerotic lesions (Vokonas & Kannel, 1996). Nonmodifiable risk factors that affect the prognosis for a person with CHD are family history, age, and gender.

The recent decline in death due to CHD are thought to be partially related to changes in lifestyle, improvement in health behavior, and improved management of atherogenic traits. Application of lifestyle changes and therapeutic interventions can lessen morbidity and mortality in older people and can be most beneficial in the high-risk elderly compared to low-risk people (Vokonas & Kannel, 1996; Wenger, 1993).

Age

The risk for CHD rises sharply with age in all populations that have been studied. The widely held belief that risk factors decrease in importance with age is inaccurate. Rather, evidence suggests that there is no age beyond which modification of risk factors will not confer a positive benefit in reduction of cardiovascular risk (Manolio et al., 1992). However, there are limited data regarding the relation between the presence of risk factors, the impact of risk modification efforts, and cardiovascular disease in older people.

In the United States, CHD becomes evident at approximately age 40, with the incidence increasing significantly after age 45 in men and 55 in women. The rate of increase in CHD mortality is linear for men, whereas in women the rate of increase is less before menopause. For women, the incidence of CHD increases rapidly following menopause. Eighty percent of all MI deaths occur in patients older than 65 years of age (Wenger, 1993).

Gender

Men continue to have a higher incidence of cardiovascular disease than women at all ages. In the United States, the age-adjusted death rates for CHD in men are twice as high as they are for women. In spite of the differences between men and women, CHD is the number one cause of death in women after age 60. Low levels of HDL-C have been identified as more of a significant predictor of CHD risk in women than in men, and in older postmenopausal women, elevated triglyceride levels have been shown to independently predict CHD risk (LaRosa & Cleeman, 1992). Women up to age 64 years are more vulnerable to risk factors of elevated systolic blood pressure, elevated blood glucose, and excess weight than are men.

Family History

CHD appears to aggregate strongly among family members. First-degree relatives of early onset CHD patients are at higher risk for developing CHD compared with the general population (Hopkins & Williams, 1989). Both genetic and environmental factors may increase family susceptibility to atherosclerosis. Genetic susceptibility has been demonstrated in animal studies and through the identification of genetic and clinical markers in humans (Hobb, Brown, & Goldstein, 1992; Williams et al., 1990). Genetic factors have been identified related to lipoprotein metabolism (LaRosa & Cleeman, 1992; Nishina, Johnson, Naggert, & Krauss, 1992). The most common syndrome found that corresponds to familial CHD is familial combined hyperlipidemia (Williams et al., 1990). Elevated fibrinogen level has been identified as an independent CHD risk factor in a number of studies (Hopkins & Williams, 1989). Environmental factors such as smoking, patterns of physical activity, and dietary intake have been significantly correlated between spouses as well as between other family members and may reflect the shared family environment (Hunt, Williams, & Barlow, 1986).

Blood Pressure and Hypertension

Hypertension is one of the most potent risk factors for all cardiovascular complications. Elevated blood pressure is the major factor underlying stroke and a major factor in MI and cardiovascular mortality. The clinical complications of hypertension result from either a direct pathologic effect on the vasculature or promotion of the atherogenic process. The risk of cardiovascular complications increases continuously with increasing levels of both systolic and diastolic blood pressure.

Hypertension is defined as sustained average blood pressure levels above 140/90 mgHg in adults. Of the 60 million Americans with hypertension, 75% have mild hypertension, or diastolic blood pressures between 90 and 105 mmHg. The term "mild" refers only to the degree of elevation and is no indication of the seriousness of the condition, because people with mild hypertension are at considerably higher risk of morbidity and mortality (Kannel, 1996). Both systolic and diastolic blood pressure are related to cardiovascular risk. People with hypertension have twice the incidence of peripheral vascular disease, sudden death, CHD, and MI and four times the incidence of stroke as those with normal blood pressure (Leon, 1991). Treatment of mild to moderate hypertension has shown significant reduction in risk for cardiovascular mortality and cerebrovascular accidents (Hebert, Moser, Mayer, Glynn, & Hennekens, 1993). A recent meta-analysis that included individuals 60 years of age and older demonstrated that antihypertensive therapy significantly improves survival and decreases stroke and cardiac mortality and morbidity (Insua et al., 1994).

Despite the clinical emphasis on diastolic hypertension, epidemiologic data substantiate the risk for CHD associated with elevations in systolic blood pressure (Vokonas, Kannel, & Cupples, 1988). Isolated systolic hypertension accounts for 65% of hypertension in older people (Joint National Committee VI, 1997).

Serum Lipids and Lipoproteins

Dyslipidemia is a major risk factor in the development and severity of CHD. Increased risk is seen in persons with elevated total cholesterol, triglycerides, LDL-C, and low levels of HDL-C. The ratio of the HDL-C fraction to the LDL-C fraction may be of greater significance than either level alone for prediction of CHD (Stampfer & Colditz, 1991). A significant positive association has been demonstrated between ingestion of dietary cholesterol, plasma cholesterol levels, and the incidence of CHD within population groups (LaRosa & Cleeman, 1992).

Longitudinal studies such as the Framingham Study and the Seven Country Study clearly demonstrate that individuals with clinical CHD have higher levels of cholesterol than do those without clinical symptoms. Prospective studies of individuals within a population have shown that serum cholesterol levels predict the future occurrence of morbidity and mortality due to CHD (Pekkanen et al., 1994).

Despite some conflicting evidence, cholesterol does appear to be a risk factor in older people (Hulley & Newman, 1994; Krumholz et al., 1994; Manolio et al., 1992). Although the direct evidence is strongest in middle-aged men with high initial cholesterol levels, epidemiologic observations support the generalization that reducing total and LDL-C levels are likely to reduce CHD incidence in older men and women and in people with more moderate elevations of cholesterol.

Lowering cholesterol levels has been shown to reduce the incidence of CHD events. It is estimated that each 1% reduction in serum cholesterol is associated with an approximate 2% reduction in coronary risk (Lipid Research Clinics Program, 1984). Similarly, each 1% increase in HDL-C has been associated with a 2% to 3% decrease in risk (Gordon et al., 1989). Two meta-analyses have shown cholesterol reduction reduced recurrent CHD events by 26% and total mortality by 9%. Angiographic studies have supported these findings by demonstrating decreased rates of progression and evidence of regression of atherosclerotic lesions in patients who lowered their LDL-C below 100 mg/dl.

The initial risk assessment based on lipid values includes measures of total cholesterol and HDL-C. The Expert Panel on Detection, Evaluation and Treatment of High Blood Cholesterol in Adults (Sempos, 1993) recommends measurement of serum total cholesterol in all adults at least once every 5 years. When assessing the risk for the elderly patient with elevated lipids, it is important to remember that the presence of known CHD, peripheral vascular, or cerebrovascular disease places the elderly patient at increased risk.

Diabetes Mellitus

Diabetes mellitus affects between 8 and 10 million Americans. Approximately 12% of those older than 65 years of age have diabetes mellitus. It is one of the leading causes of disability in those older than 45 years of age. CHD represents the ultimate cause of death in more than half of diabetic patients and tends to occur at an earlier age and with greater severity than in the nondiabetic population.

Accelerated atherosclerosis is a major complication of diabetes mellitus. Accelerated atherogenesis may be related to factors such as hyperglycemia, hyperinsulinemia, and plasma lipid abnormalities, all of which are common in diabetics. Data demonstrate that risk factors for CHD tend to "cluster" in diabetic patients. Patients with diabetes are more likely to be obese, have abnormal lipid profiles, and are more likely to be hypertensive. Hyperglycemia is considered to be an independent risk factor in the development of CHD in diabetics. Increased blood glucose is associated with increased plasma lipid levels, elevated mean systolic and diastolic blood pressures, and a higher mean body mass. Accelerated atherosclerosis in patients with diabetes mellitus indicates an alteration in both lipid and lipoprotein metabolism. Elevation of VLDL-C concentrations occurs frequently in insulin-dependent diabetics, resulting in increased total plasma cholesterol and triglyceride levels.

The relation between glycemic control and plasma cholesterol and triglyceride levels may be significant in altering the predicted risk of CHD in non-insulin-dependent diabetics. Although both male and female non-insulin-dependent diabetics have lower HDL-C levels than do nondiabetic controls, the relative decrease is greater for women (Levy & Kannel, 1988). Another potential risk factor for CHD in the diabetic is the level of circulating insulin. Hyperinsulinemia promotes ischemic vascular disease and is a risk factor independent of the blood glucose level, plasma cholesterol, and blood pressure. Because hyperinsulinemia characterizes the initial stages of type II diabetes, individuals may be exposed to increased circulating insulin levels over time. Hyperinsulinemia is prevalent in type II diabetics secondary to insulin resistance related to obesity.

Psychosocial and Contextual Factors

The incidence of CHD cannot be completely explained by the major CHD risk factors. Considerable evidence suggests that psychosocial and environmental factors may be independent predictors of CHD incidence in population studies (Orth-Gomer, Rosengren, & Wilhelmsen, 1993; Wamala, Wolk, Schenck-Gustafsson, & Orth-Gomer, 1997). These factors include coronary-prone behavior and aspects of the social context.

Coronary-Prone Behavior

Several studies have identified type A behavior pattern, which includes time urgency and competitiveness, as a risk factor for CHD. Data from the Framingham study suggest that women with type A personalities are at increased risk for the development of heart disease (Haynes & Feinleib, 1980). However, the relation between type A behavior pattern and CHD morbidity and mortality continues to be debated. Some evidence indicates that anger and hostility components may be more important predictors of cardiovascular outcome (Williams, 1987). The ability to express anger may be of particular importance in women (Eaker, 1989). More recent studies document a significant relation between hostility and perfusion defects among women and middle-aged men (Helmers et al., 1993).

Social Context

Lower SES has been documented as a factor associated with increased CHD mortality in both men and women. Research examining the relations between behavioral risk factors for CHD and socioeconomic characteristics has identified direct relations between the practice of risk-reducing behaviors and level of income, education, and occupational status (Wing, Casper, Riggan, Hayes, & Tyroler, 1988).

Low levels of social support, weak social connections, and social isolation have been consistently related to adverse health outcomes. Social support has been associated with decreased cardiac mortality, enhanced physical and psychosocial function, and adherence to risk modification (Dracup, 1994; Moser, 1994; Riegel, 1989). Social isolation has been consistently associated with an increase in mortality rates from CHD (Berkman & Seeman, 1986; Seeman & Syme, 1987). Elderly identified to be at highest risk for mortality from CHD are those who live alone and are socially isolated. Researchers have reported that socially isolated women with high amounts of life stress experienced four times the risk of death from CHD than those with low life stress and less limited socialization (Lyness et al., 1996).

POLYPHARMACY

High rates of prescription medication use and the concurrent use of several drugs among older adults correspond to the prevalence of acute and chronic illness in this population. Older people use more prescription and nonprescription drugs than do younger people and often require a number of medications. Adults aged 65 and older make up 12% of the population and have been found to use 30% of all prescription medication. Nonprescription drug use among older people is approximately seven times that of the general population. Chrischilles, Segar, and Wallace (1992) found that between 60% and 78% of community-dwelling elders used at least one prescription drug. The average community-dwelling elder takes one prescription drug and three over-the-counter drugs on a regular basis (Moellar & Mathiowetz, 1989). This high rate of polypharmacy places elders at risk for potentially serious physical and behavioral adverse drug reactions (Burke, Jolson, Goetsch, & Ahronheim, 1992; Hartshorn & Tatro, 1991; Ray, Griffin, & Shorr, 1990; Vestal, 1990). A direct relation has been noted between the number of drugs taken and the risk of adverse effects in older people (Rho & Wong, 1998). The health risks associated with polypharmacy as well as the high cost of medications emphasize the importance of effective drug treatment that addresses the number of medications prescribed, complexity, and cost of medication regimens for older people.

Adverse effects in older people may reflect the potential for adverse drug interactions with the use of multiple medications, failure to take medications according to the dosage and timing prescribed, and changes in the pharmodynamics of drug use (Brummel-Smith, 1998). Age-related changes in cognitive function and failing vision may cause elders to make mistakes in the dosage of medication taken. Furthermore, multiple disease processes, slowed metabolism, and decreases in renal and hepatic function reduce clearance of medication, leading to increased medication side effects in many elderly. Increases in the proportion of body fat and decreases in the proportion of body water that occur with aging may predispose older people to a high level of fat-soluble medications in adipose tissue and increases in the concentration of hydrophilic medications in the blood.

The behavioral manifestations of adverse drug effects among older people include depression, confusion, sedation, and functional impairment (Larson, Kukull, Buchner, & Reifler, 1987). The effects of drugs—particularly benzodiazepines, barbiturates, and antidepressants—are among the most common causes of falls in older people (Herings, Stricker, de Boer, Bakker, & Sturmans, 1995; Rubenstein, 1998). These outcomes are found even with many commonly used drugs, emphasizing the need for caution in prescribing and monitoring even routine medication use among older adults (Vestal & Dawson, 1985).

HORMONE ALTERATIONS AT MIDLIFE

Health Consequences of Menopause

Mean life expectancy for U.S. women now exceeds 84 years (Scharbo-Dehaan, 1996). Menopause typically occurs at the average age of 51, with women living one third of their lives following menopause (Kaiser, Wilson, & Morley, 1997). Ovarian follicles, numbering 200,000 to 300,000 at puberty, decline with age. The ovary becomes shrunken and fibrotic; ova and follicles disappear (Kaiser et al., 1997). By age 45, there are approximately 8,000 follicles left (Kaiser et al., 1997). Without follicles, the ovary does not produce sufficient amounts of estrogen; without estrogen stimulation of the endometrium, menopause and associated symptoms occur (Soules & Bremner, 1982). Estrone becomes the major circulating estrogen; production of the androgen dehydroepiandrosterone and its sulfate remain unchanged, creating an alteration in the estrogen-androgen ratio. The estrogen component is lower, the androgen component higher (Kaiser et al., 1997).

Vasomotor changes, experienced as hot flashes or flushes, are a major symptom of the perimenopause. These symptoms are identical to those that occur with central activation of heat loss mechanisms (Mashchak, Kletzky, Artal, & Mishell, 1984). These troubling symptoms virtually disappear over time and are not a problem among most older women. However, following menopause, an increase in the release of interleukins (IL) from monocytes occurs (Breder et al., 1988). IL-1 is a recognized pyrogen; elevated levels can produce pathphysiologic changes similar to the hot flash, and this can occur at any older age.

Changes in estrogen ratio affect the balance of several body systems. Uterine size is decreased due to myometrial atrophy, the vaginal vault becomes shortened, rugal folds are lost, and there is thinning of the vaginal mucosa (Kaiser et al., 1997). Many women experience vaginal dryness and vaginitis, which may, in turn, lead to dyspareunia and loss of sexual desire (Lichtman, 1996). A variety of additional symptoms occur in estrogen-dependent urogenital structures, leading to urinary incontinence and cystitis in the older woman (Kaiser et al., 1997).

Headaches and insomnia may be experienced, along with changes in the cognitive domain such as loss of concentration, loss of memory, mood changes, and depression (Avis, Brambilla, McKinaly, & Vass, 1994; Stewart & Boydell, 1993). Estrogen depletion has major effects on the cardiovascular system, influencing lipid and lipoprotein levels, blood pressure, and carbohydrate metabolism (PEPI Writing Group, 1995). Lower estrogen levels contribute to an acceleration of bone loss in older women. Following the menopause, women experience a change in regional fat distribution, with fat depots becoming more centrally distributed (Ley, Lees, & Stevenson, 1992; Shimokata et al., 1989). Some investigators suggest that the unfavorable fat distribution in women is more dependent on age than on menopause (Wang, Hassager, Ravn, Wang, & Christiansen, 1994). However, the postmenopausal decline in fat-free mass (lean tissue mass and bone mass) are menopausal-related (Wang et al., 1994).

PSYCHOSOCIAL RISKS IN OLDER PEOPLE

Although longevity has increased, multiple mental health challenges and stresses can characterize the quality of life in later years. Old age is associated with many life changes, including changing physical and mental abilities, changing social roles, loss of spouse or close friends, and changes in lifestyle and economic resources (Kaplan, 1997).

The stresses associated with aging may take a significant toll on the health and productive functioning of older adults. It is important to establish mental health promotion for sustained vitality and productivity in late adulthood. Equally important, we need to understand the large individual differences among older adults in responding to the stresses and challenges of later life. Among the most common problems of older people are depression and sleep disorders, as well as a challenging physical and social environment. These risks may affect the underlying physical illness, cause substantial mental distress, and increase the costs of care.

Depression

Among mental health disorders in late life, depression is common (Anthony & Aboraya, 1992) and is often underrecognized and undertreated among older adults (Borchelt & Horgas, 1994). It is thought that nearly 5 million individuals age 65 and over suffer from serious and persistent symptoms of depression, and more than 1 million suffer from major depression. However, the exact prevalence of depression in late life is unclear because reports vary widely depending on the definition and methodology used (Staudinger, Marsiske, & Baltes, 1993).

Depression is a clinical syndrome that affects older adults in a variety of ways. Depressive symptoms and disorders are associated with social withdrawal, isolation, physical complaints, and functional decline (Cohen, 1990), all of which can contribute to physical and behavioral dependency. Depression is one of the most common causes of "failure to thrive" in older people and may initiate the multiple consequences of functional disability and immobility (Robinson, 1998). Most of the treatment for older adults' depression occurs in the context of a primary care medical practice, with only a small minority of depressed older adults being treated by a mental health practitioner. Thus, depression among older adults often goes undetected and untreated, eroding the quality of life and productivity of older adults.

The origins of depression among older people are thought to be related to biological factors, physical factors, psychological processes, and social influences (Muller-Spahn & Hock, 1994). Biological processes may reflect genetic influences, changes in neurophysiology, and disruption of biological patterns with age. Depressive symptoms often are influenced by the psychobiological changes that occur with aging and place older people at greater risk for a depressive disorder with biological origins (Blazer, 1993). Physical and psychological factors include response to specific disease processes, side effects of medication, and sensory changes. An inability to adapt successfully to the physical and social changes that occur with aging may contribute to depression in older people (Blazer, 1993). Related social factors include changes in social relationships, social isolation, and a decrease in needed social support. Challenges in later life include changes in valued social roles, decreased economic resources, and the loss of loved ones.

Sleep Disorders

Sleep and aging literature largely support the conclusions that with aging the ability to sleep diminishes, but the need for sleep does not. Sleep disturbances, including difficulty in falling asleep, frequent awakenings during the night, early morning awakenings, or complaints of poor-quality sleep are common concerns among older people. Data have shown that older adults frequently experience nighttime waking and that many routinely use sleep medication. Sleep pattern disturbance reflects an alteration in the elderly person's habitual pattern of sleep and wakefulness that causes discomfort or interferes with a desired lifestyle. Functional problems associated with sleep deprivation include difficulty with memory, concentration, and motor skills. Additional problems include increased aggressiveness and irritability and neurological disturbances (Bootzin, Epstein, Engle-Friedman, & Salvio, 1995).

Physical and Social Environment

Characteristics of the physical and social environment have been implicated in how older people respond to biological aging and health promotion efforts. Properties of the physical and social environment clearly have an impact on the health of aged persons, but there have been few attempts to examine the extent of the impact.

Most older persons "grow old in place," that is, they remain in the same communities, churches, often in the same house that they have occupied for most of their adult lives. However, for many older people, housing and community resources may become unsatisfactory over time. As people live longer and experience extended periods of frailty, many older people find it difficult to age in place. Because safe and adequate shelter is a basic human need, housing problems may significantly affect the health of the elderly person. Those in substandard housing are at higher risk for poor outcomes in health and have higher demands placed on an already strained reserve of resources. Inadequate housing may contribute to health problems such as falls, social isolation, and poverty (Kaplan, 1997). It has been estimated that environmental hazards, in the context of intrinsic limitations, play a role in one third to one half of all home falls (Hornbrook et al., 1994). According to Kendig (1990), the primary housing-related problem for older adults is inadequacy of housing for an individual's needs. Redfoot and Gaberlavage (1991) found those housing quality problems are most frequent among (a) minority elders, (b) single-person households, (c) rural elders, and (d) central city dwellers.

For some older adults, homes and neighborhoods begin to deteriorate over time and become unsafe living environments. In other cases, elders are no longer able to live alone. Attempts to relocate to improved housing or assisted-living facilities may not be possible due to high costs or limited availability of affordable housing (Aday, 1993). With limited economic resources, the older person may be forced to remain in community, where a risk of crime and violence toward them exists.

Properties of the physical environment have some impact on the health of aged persons, but there have been few attempts to examine these properties and their impact on the elderly community (Balsam & Bottum, 1997). Environmental factors can have an indirect effect on health through the limits placed on health promotion behaviors in the community. The design of housing and neighborhoods, outdoor lighting, and the perception of safety might affect levels of physical activity, social contact, and support provided.

CHAPTER 3

Theoretical Models for Health Promotion in Older People

S eeking, developing, and using theoretical models for risk reduction and health promotion efforts in older people require thoughtful consideration of several issues. These include the purpose and function of theoretical approaches, their pragmatic relevance in health behavior change, and their usefulness in guiding subsequent clinical investigations. Theoretical models may be effective guides to research and practice and as a guide for the development of interventions that improve the health of the public (Freudenberg et al., 1995). Theoretical models that are relevant to the health of the public must be able to describe why a particular kind of intervention will lead to the desired outcome (Freudenberg et al., 1995).

Several changes in health issues and in the U.S. population have stimulated the need for rational, theoretically based interventions directed toward health promotion. First, the concept of illness has changed dramatically (Freudenberg et al., 1995). Acute and chronic illnesses are increasingly recognized as lifestyle disease, directly related to patterns of initiation and maintenance in health promotion and disease prevention behavior. Social problems, such as drug use and violence, are now considered chronic in nature. Theoretical models and health education interventions need to focus on individual and community lifestyle changes that address the prevention of acute and chronic illness (Freundenberg et al., 1995).

There is increasing diversity among the people of the United States, along with remarkable within-culture and within-ethnic group variation. This requires that theoretical approaches to health promotion interventions examine cultural sensitivity and specificity among groups targeted for health promotion interventions. There is a significant relation between economic status and health status, along with a gap in health outcomes between the rich and the poor. This requires that health promotion efforts become acceptable and accessible to a wide variety of socioeconomic and sociocultural groups.

Many efforts designed to address health promotion in older people have focused on strategies for reducing health risk, including both individual lifestyle change and community or system-wide change. An individual approach identifies a finite number of lifestyle areas that can be targeted for intervention. Individual lifestyle change alters the choices individuals make about their health without changing the environment in which choices are made. Community-based approaches strive to create supportive environments within which health choices are facilitated (Flynn, Rider, & Ray, 1991). In a community-based approach, systems represent the social, political, institutional, cultural, legislative, and physical environment in which health behavior occurs.

INDIVIDUAL-LEVEL MODELS

The majority of models created to explain and predict efforts to reduce health risk in older people have defined such efforts as a personal matter, one in which the individual has an obligation. Models of health behavior change currently proposed and used as a basis for clinical research and practice have been derived from social cognitive theory and include the Health Belief Model (Maimen & Becker, 1974), the Theory of Reasoned Action (Ajzen & Fishbein, 1980), Self-Efficacy Theory (Bandura, 1986, 1997), the Relapse Prevention Model (Marlatt & Gordon, 1985), and the Transtheoretical Model (Prochaska & DiClemente, 1984).

The Health Belief Model (HBM) is a cognitive behavioral model that was developed in an attempt to predict when people will engage in preventive behaviors (Maimen & Becker, 1974). Developed to explain health-related behavior in terms of subjective beliefs, the HBM focuses on individual cognition or perceptions of the present environment (Rosenstock, 1974). The HBM has been used primarily to describe individually focused behavioral outcomes rather than to guide interventions as a model. The four core dimensions of the HBM—susceptibility, severity, benefits, and barriers—have been applied in many studies over the past 40 years in an attempt to explain and predict cardiovascular risk factor reduction in men and women, including smoking cessation, regular physical activity, and antihypertensive therapy.

Across studies using the HBM as a theoretical framework, individual perception of barriers has been most consistently associated with health-promoting behaviors. Perceived susceptibility to illness and perceived severity of health outcomes have contributed significantly to health-promoting behavior related to smoking cessation, adherence to an antihypertensive medication regimen, and participation in programs of regular physical activity.

Self-Efficacy Theory (Bandura, 1986) incorporates beliefs about individual outcomes and efficacy expectations. Outcome expectations are beliefs about whether a behavior will lead to a certain outcome. Efficacy expectations are beliefs about one's competence to perform a behavior that will lead to the expected results. The self-efficacy concept has been most commonly applied to cardiovascular health promotion interventions, including smoking behaviors, weight control, and physical activity, with varying levels of success. Studies investigating individual health behavior using Self-Efficacy Theory have found a sense of mastery and competence to be an important factor in the individual decision to initiate health promotion behaviors.

The Theory of Reasoned Action (TRA) focuses on an individual's intention to undertake behavior change (Ajzen & Fishbein, 1980). The major dimensions of the model—attitudes and subjective norms or perceived social pressure—determine the intention to engage in a particular behavior. The TRA hypothesizes that individuals are more likely to take action or change behavior if they believe their actions will lead to desired outcomes. In addition, subjective norms, or the pressure of significant others' feelings about the need for the individual to change, motivate the individual to change behavior. The theory has been applied to individual decision making related to the initiation of regular physical activity, weight loss, smoking cessation, and stress management. Research using the TRA as a theoretical framework supports the attitudinal dimension of intent as a primary predictor of health promotion efforts.

The Relapse Prevention Model (RPM; Marlatt & Gordon, 1985) was designed initially to explain abstinence from cigarette smoking and substance abuse. The RPM includes an analysis of lifestyle imbalances, dissonance, positive outcome expectancies for relapse, high-risk situations for relapse, and abstinence violation. In a retrospective examination of lifetime history of relapse from physical activity in healthy adults, Sallis and Hovell (1990) reported that 20% of participants had experienced three or more relapses in regular physical activity. Krug, Haire-Joshu, and Heady (1991) found that 70% of diabetic patients surveyed reported a relapse during attempts to establish physical activity, and 64% reported two or more relapse episodes. Intervention studies based on the RPM have shown variable effectiveness, with high attrition in some studies (Belisle, Roskies, & Levesque, 1987; King, Taylor, Haskell, & Debusk, 1988; Marcus, Selby, Niaura, & Rossi, 1992). The complete RPM has not been tested or validated related to health promotion behavior. Despite the potential for relapse prevention concepts to increase our understanding of addictive behavior, it is not known whether RPM concepts may be applied in the same ways to the maintenance of healthy behaviors or health promotion efforts.

The Transtheoretical Model (TTM; DiClemente & Prochaska, 1983) proposes that two interrelated dimensions are needed to assess behavior modification adequately: (a) stages of change, which represent the temporal, motivational, and constancy aspects of change; and (b) processes of change, which focus on activities and events that create successful modification of a problem behavior. A strength of the model is its focus on the dynamic nature of health behavior change. Research examining stages of change in healthy individuals has identified significant differences in activity levels, outcome beliefs (Sonstroem & Morgan, 1989), and determinants of activity acquisition (Marcus, Rossi, Selby, Niaura, & Abrams, 1992) among participants in different stages of change. The effectiveness of intervention studies based on the TTM has varied across studies with healthy adults (Cardinal & Sachs, 1996; Lombard, Lombard, & Winett, 1995; Marcus, Rossi, et al., 1992). Applicability of the TTM as a predictive model or as a basis for intervention has not been examined in elderly individuals or in lifestyle changes. Furthermore, model variables associated with stages of change differ across studies and have provided only limited examination of interventions directed toward long-term behavioral change (Marcus, Selby, et al., 1992).

Theories of behavior change have focused on mechanisms for increasing the level of preparedness to change, improving motivation to change, learning the skills necessary for change, and maintaining new behaviors (Carleton & Lasater, 1994). These models have yielded significant though inconsistent results in explaining and predicting individual adherence in initiating and maintaining health behavior. The variability of findings using cognitive behavioral theories suggests that there may be more to health promotion efforts than can be explained by individual attitudes and beliefs alone. Many health behavior models are based on the framework and assumption that individuals can change their health outcomes simply by altering their lifestyle. Individual lifestyle changes have significant merit but fail to explain how cultural and structural aspects of the elder's place in society impinge on their health status.

Individual models attempt to explain and predict behavioral change but do not address the development of community competencies in the achievement of health promotion risk reduction. Rather, the focus is on addressing individual weakness and attempts to motivate change from a deficit perspective (Eng, Salmon, & Mullan, 1992). There is limited exploration of how attitudes and health beliefs may change in relation to life events, or exploration of the role of modifying factors—including minimal resources, educational level, and access to resources—in determining health outcomes. The majority of prospective investigations have not demonstrated significant relations between individual variables when initiating a program of health behavior and sustained adherence, compared with relations between model variables and concurrent health behavior.

It appears that the values elderly individuals hold regarding health matters and their perceptions of control over their health affect health-related decisions more than do individual motivation factors. For example, Bandura's Self-Efficacy Theory, along with Kanfer's model of self-control and self-change, was used to examine health behavior changes in a group of Medicare recipients (Elder, Williams, Drew, Wright, & Boulan, 1995). These Medicare participants (N = 1,800) were randomized into two groups: usual care (control) and preventive care (theory-based intervention). The theory-based intervention was based on self-efficacy and emphasized goal setting, individual counseling, and problem solving. Although changes in the physical activity of the intervention group were sustained over time (2 years), it was difficult to determine whether the interventions targeted toward self-efficacy enhancement were responsible. However, certain individual variables were affected: Perceptions of self-control over health matters were substantially greater in the intervention group, and physical activity behavior changes were realized through goal setting and counseling (Elder et al., 1995). Results from the Rancho Bernardo Heart and Chronic Disease Survey demonstrated a positive and significant relation between individual health beliefs and self-reported health behavior change (Ferrini, Edelstein, & Barrett-Connor, 1994). Respondents in that study with positive health beliefs concerning the value of diet and exercise in health promotion efforts were more likely to report positive changes in health behavior (Ferrini et al., 1994).

Individual models have often failed to consider issues of relevance to elders, including differences in disease progression and symptomology as well as specific environmental factors, such as role strain, occupational stresses, or lack of resources (Srebnik, 1991). The influence of interpersonal, environmental, and cultural factors on health behavior are not addressed. Ongoing efforts include the need to test the individual models across socioeconomic, racial, and ethnic groups, because little or no emphasis has been placed on the influence of these factors in lifestyle development and change.

The application of individual models to persons of varying socioeconomic and educational backgrounds also needs further development and testing (Haber, 1996). Certain groups of older people may have differing perspectives of the health care system, which may affect their willingness to participate in individually focused risk reduction efforts. For example, older African Americans may have experienced years of racial discrimination and may be less trusting of the health care system, health education, and scientific data. Older people of limited educational attainment may be ill equipped to comprehend or use health information (Haber, 1996). Rural elders may lack access to health promotion activities and materials due to geographical isolation and a lack of community resources.

Given the difficulties identified in predicting determinants of motivation and in assisting older people in sustained risk modification, it may be unrealistic to rely on individual behavioral change alone to reduce the burden of illness (Cominellis, 1993). Models that focus primarily on individual lifestyle changes most often do not take into account external, societal factors or attempt to effect change within a broader social context (Srebnik, 1991). Efforts designed to address the social contextual elements of health promotion and disease prevention in older people must begin to more closely examine those aspects of the individual in the community as a basis for prevention.

COMMUNITY-BASED MODELS

Community psychologists have suggested that health promotion efforts move beyond a focus on individual lifestyle change to the creation of supportive environments in which healthy living can take place (Green & Kreuter, 1990). Consistent with these trends, the concept of community as a physical setting has been redefined to focus on community as a living being with interactive ties among organizations, neighborhoods, families, and friends. It may refer to a geographic community, cultural community, or societal community. The emphasis in health promotion and disease prevention at the community level is on an integrated, person-environment approach in which the responsibility for heath is shared between individuals and systems. As such, the health of the community is directly related to the health of its members (Eng et al., 1992). A number of community-based models have been developed and tested for the prevention of coronary heart disease (CHD). Large-scale trials have attempted to implement community action and social change by altering social structures, facilitating community empowerment, and through communication and media marketing strategies (Murdaugh & Vanderboom, 1997).

The ecological framework for community-based intervention presents a perspective for defining health and human behavior, positing that although people will choose to take health action on the basis of need, not all people have the same opportunities for choosing (Eng et al., 1992). The range of intervention options is widened from an exclusive focus on changing individuals' knowledge, attitudes, and practices to exploring the development of community competence. From an ecological perspective, additional intervention options include changing conditions in the social environment created by groups, organizations, and communities and policies that influence individuals' health and behaviors. This perspective provides a framework for defining problems and determining multiple levels of intervention driven by an imperative to increase community competence.

Social ecology supports the creation of health promotion activities that are agreed on and developed by community members along with the development of health-promoting public policy (Stokols, 1992, 1996) and communication focused on the diffusion of innovation (Rogers, 1995). Common to all successful attempts at community-based intervention are the critical elements of community organization (leadership), community settings (work, church, school), and a focus on environmental change (Flynn et al., 1991).

Examples of community-based intervention projects that incorporate the ecological view of health and the sociopolitical context in health promotion include the North Karelia Project in Finland (Puska, Nissinen, Tuomilehto, Saloven, & Koskela, 1985), the Stanford Three Community Study (Fortmann, Williams, Hulley, Haskell, & Farquhar, 1981), the Stanford Five City Research Project (Farquhar, Fortmann, Flora, Taylor, & Haskell, 1990), the Minnesota Heart Health Program (Luepker et al., 1985), and Healthy Cities Indiana (Flynn et al., 1991). Projects have emphasized community leadership development in health promotion; a unified voice for health; and improvement in community life, services, and resources.

The North Karelia Project was a multifaceted, community-based intervention using the media, trained local personnel, community organization approaches, and health care professionals to influence population behaviors, risk factors, and morbidity and mortality. The Stanford Three Community Study used electronic media, supplemented in one community by individualized counseling in a 2-year intervention program designed to influence risk factors but not to measure disease prevalence (Fortmann et al., 1981). The Five City Research Project expanded this effort to include the use of electronic and print media, individual and group counseling, and involvement of diverse groups in the intervention communities. In the Minnesota Heart Health Program, influential community leaders served on community advisory boards in the three intervention communities. The media were used less than in the Stanford program, and population-based risk factor screening and direct counseling were more prominent. Parents and children were taught about smoking prevention and other risk reductions in schools and work sites and throughout the communities. As a model still developing, the Healthy Cities process includes city commitment, community leadership development, city action, provision of data-based information to policymakers, and action research and evaluation.

Community empowerment is defined as the process by which communities predict, control, and participate in developing their own health environment (Minkler, 1990). The empowerment process enables community members to gain control over their lives in the context of changing their environment. At the community level, empowerment is often referred to as "community competence," because empowered communities are capable of solving their own problems (Levine & Perkins, 1997; Wallerstein & Bernstein, 1994). Community empowerment begins when community members engage simultaneously as teachers and learners to listen to each other and begin to communicate to develop strategies for change. Elements of empowerment that must be incorporated into successful health promotion program development have been identified (Wallerstein, 1992). The program needs to build in the opportunity to share ideas and concerns and develop trust. Program leaders assume the role of facilitators and problem posers instead of directors and problem solvers.

The Pawtucket Heart Health Program (Assaf, Banspach, & Laster, 1987), the Heart, Body and Soul Project (Robbins, 1991), the Five a Day for Better Health Program (Baranowski, 1995), and the Heart to Heart Project (Goodman, Wheeler, & Lee, 1995) represent community-based programs that have promoted community competence through the use of empowerment. Across projects, community members expressed the relevant needs and interests of the community, existing resources in the community were identified to clarify gaps in services and resources, and community members were provided consultation to implement the interventions. Interventions have included physical fitness campaigns, smoking cessation efforts, and "shop smart" campaigns. Project activities include health fair screenings and educational programs. Programs have promoted community ownership through the use of volunteers in church-based interventions and have included work sites, schools, and government agencies, as well as the use of multidisciplinary teams with members from academic, governmental, private sector, and volunteer agencies.

Community-based models incorporate elements that influence health beyond individual attitudes and beliefs, to target the system in which individuals live and work. The models presented attempt community-based change by acknowledging the person-in-context. This systems perspective for prevention mandates a united purpose at many levels to implement change (Stokols, 1996). Although researchers did attempt to "share" the change process with participating communities, it is not clear the extent to which the community-based interventions presented included all community members as equal partners. Many of the communities targeted were white and middle class, limiting our understanding of diverse perspectives, including those of the disenfranchised, minority groups, and women in poverty.

Community-based interventions did include competency enhancement in the prevention of chronic health problems, such as CHD, but they were not specific in the extent to which they explored and addressed the concerns of older people in the community, particularly the underserved and minority elderly. There was little attention to socioeconomic and psychological issues, including access to health care, material resources, work environment, or role strain. Programs targeted specific, traditional risk factors for intervention rather than examining risk as including socioeconomic and environmental factors. For example, educational programs teaching individuals how to shop for low-fat foods may be one method of preventing chronic illness, but they do not take into account the needs of those with limited resources. Few of the interventions attempted to address issues of service systems, political action, or the rights of older people as citizens.

Several major weaknesses accompany the cited successes of community health promotion programs. The first is the issue of generalizability. These first-generation demonstration projects had large budgets; the challenge for the empowerment of groups and communities is to initiate health promotion programs that have realistic budgets and that involve state and community leadership and resources (Elder et al., 1995). Second, little effort for intervention was placed on low income, inner-city, or minority populations (Elder et al., 1995). It is these groups that are the most vulnerable to social inequity of resources and discrimination in health matters. Projects that have targeted minority groups have not documented the success of other community-based heart health projects. The Physical Activity for Risk Reduction project (Luepker et al., 1985) and other center-based programs have found low participation rates; conflicts with work and failure to reach the hard-to-reach were cited among other reasons for poor participation (Baranowski, 1995; Lewis et al., 1993).

A third major weakness of even those successful community-based interventions has been the failure to acknowledge secular trends in economic development that influence lifestyle decisions. For example, there have been changes in societal patterns of physical activity. Work for many individuals is sedentary, insecure, and mechanized, all of which affects the work stress and sedentary behavior that contributes to health risk.

In summary, theoretical models to guide the development and implementation of health promotion interventions are needed. Individual models, particularly the more salient characteristics within those models such as "barriers" and "self-efficacy," have demonstrated significant relations to the engagement in health promotion behavior. However, the complexity of health promotion efforts—including societal barriers such as poverty, access to health care, transportation, and isolation—require more community-based efforts. Combining characteristics inherent in individual models with community engagement strategies may be the critical element needed to focus on individual and community-level change needed for healthy elders.

CHAPTER 4

Health Promotion Interventions

SMOKING CESSATION

The cessation rate among U.S. adults who have ever smoked varies by age, gender, education, race, and geography. Despite knowledge of the adverse health consequences of smoking, one third of the adults in the United States continue to smoke. For millions of adults, efforts to quit smoking have failed (U.S. Department of Health and Human Services [USDHHS], 1991). Individual and community-based interventions need to begin by making smokers aware of the consequences of smoking as well as the benefits of quitting. Even after the age of 60, smoking cessation has been shown to lead to improved pulmonary function.

Smoking cessation is accompanied by a number of symptoms consistent with withdrawal. Withdrawal symptoms—including nicotine craving, irritability, frustration, anxiety, restlessness, and difficulty concentrating—may appear as soon as 2 hours after cessation and may persist for a variable period of time. The intensity of these symptoms, particularly the craving for nicotine, can undermine even a strong commitment to smoking cessation. People who smoke more than one pack of cigarettes per day or who have their first cigarette of the day within 10 minutes of waking are more likely to experience a greater magnitude in symptoms immediately following cessation (Becker et al., 1993). Other symptoms associated with smoking cessation include sleep disturbances and gastrointestinal symptoms. Although these withdrawal symptoms generally improve within a few weeks, they may undermine sustained cessation efforts. An increase in coughing may be noted initially as some of the paralytic effects of smoking on mucociliary function are reversed. After nicotine withdrawal and its physiological symptoms have diminished, patients still must face the loss of a pharmacological agent they may have used to cope with many of life's stresses and demands.

Pharmacological Interventions

A number of forms of pharmacotherapy have been used and are being evaluated for the treatment of cigarette smoking. Nicotine is known to be the dependence-producing substance in tobacco. Nicotine easily crosses the blood-brain barrier to affect both mood and cognitive function. For this reason, nicotine substitution therapy has been a successful pharmacological approach to smoking cessation. The goal of nicotine replacement is to provide smokers with the primary pharmacological reinforcement of smoking—nicotine—to reduce physical withdrawal symptoms after smoking cessation. Relief from or reduction of withdrawal symptoms can improve initial abstinence rates and may improve long-term abstinence (Fiore, Kenford, et al., 1994). Although studies that have included elderly smokers are limited, nicotine replacement combined with behavioral training has been shown to be effective (Fiore, Smith, Jorenby, & Baker, 1994; Silagy, Mant, Fowler, & Lodge, 1994).

Recently, recognition of the difficulty involved in smoking cessation has raised questions about the adequacy of the traditional emphasis on abstinence as the only therapeutic goal (Warner, Slade, & Sweanor, 1997). A harm-reduction strategy has been proposed that includes extended nicotine maintenance without the harmful substances found in tobacco (Hughes, 1995).

Guidelines for smoking cessation from the Agency for Health Care Policy and Research (AHCPR) recommend the use of the nicotine patch for routine clinical use due to issues of adherence and patient training. Nicotine replacement therapy via a transdermal delivery system has demonstrated effectiveness in all but patients with unstable ischemic heart disease. Clinical trials of transdermal nicotine replacement indicate that this therapy can be effective, with initial cessation rates of 25% to 80% (Buchkremer, Minneker, & Block, 1991; Tonnesen, Norregaard, Simonson, & Sawe, 1992), and cessation rates between 12% and 35% at the end of 1 to 2 years. However, symptom relief during withdrawal may require an individualized patch dosage designed to achieve adequate blood levels of nicotine. For patients who continue to smoke following 2 weeks of patch therapy, transdermal patch therapy should be discontinued and a new quit date set (Fiore, 1994). Higher doses of nicotine using the transdermal patch as well as mechanisms for dose titration are being examined to provide optimum nicotine replacement. Although use of a

44-mg patch dose appears to be safe (Henningfield et al., 1992), the efficacy of higher doses of nicotine in improving cessation rates is not known. Studies have demonstrated the efficacy of transdermal patch therapy during active treatment (Fiore, 1992), and a fall in cessation rates following treatment has been noted. Relapse following pharmacological therapy emphasizes the importance of continued support, counseling regarding coping strategies, and overcoming barriers to sustained behavioral change. Few systemic side effects have been noted with patch use. Skin reactions have been reported frequently, with itching and redness at patch sites occurring in up to 50% of patch users (Fiore, 1992).

Nicotine replacement therapy using nicotine gum has been a successful pharmacological approach to smoking cessation. Nicotine gum may be most effective when used to supplement a comprehensive smoking cessation program. When nicotine gum is used regularly throughout the day, the levels of nicotine average one third to two thirds of the levels observed with cigarette smoking. The use of nicotine chewing gum has shown a success rate in smoking cessation of approximately 23% at 6 months, declining to 11% at 1 year (Buchkremer et al., 1991; Tonnesen et al., 1992). However, a number of studies have found no significant improvement in smoking cessation for nicotine versus placebo gum treatment when combined with physician intervention (Cohen et al., 1989; Hughes, 1996).

Nicotine gum reduces nicotine withdrawal symptoms and provides a substitute oral activity. The lack of effectiveness noted using this pharmacological therapy may be due, in part, to poor patient adherence in the use of gum or interfered nicotine absorption due to changes in salivary pH (Henningfield, 1990). Side effects of nicotine gum include hiccups, sore throat, and gastrointestinal symptoms such as nausea. Patients who experience side effects should be instructed to chew the gum more slowly.

Although not addressed in the AHCPR guidelines, nicotine nasal spray recently has become available as a prescription drug, and a nicotine inhaler has been approved for marketing by the U.S. Food and Drug Administration (Lunell, Molander, Leischow, & Fagerstrom, 1995). Data available on these products indicate that the nicotine nasal spray and inhaler are as effective as nicotine gum and the nicotine patch (Hjalmarson, Franzon, Westin, & Wiklund, 1994). The antidepressant drug buproprion has been approved as pharmacotherapy for smoking cessation.

Two common problems often diminish the effectiveness of nicotine replacement. The first is the expectation that it is a cure that will remove all symptoms. Nicotine replacement is an adjunct treatment, and other behavioral and cognitive treatments are extremely important. Nicotine replacement should be used for a number of months. For patients chewing the gum, weaning may be achieved by means of a fixed tapering schedule, or the patient may reduce the amount slowly according to symptoms. For those using the dermal patches, the prescribed stepped regimen automatically tapers the dose. Nicotine replacement therapy must be used with caution in persons with severe hypertension, arrhythmia, unstable angina, or recent myocardial infarction, because it has been shown to increase both heart rate and blood pressure.

Behavioral and Cognitive Interventions

The American Heart Association (1998) Consensus Panel advised that patients with cardiovascular disease and their families be strongly advised to stop smoking. Patients must be provided with counseling, nicotine replacement, and formal cessation programs as part of appropriate strategies for reduction of the risks associated with cigarette smoking. An array of behavioral, cognitive, psychodynamic, and educational methods for smoking cessation exist and may be used alone or in combination with pharmacological therapy. Each method offers some benefit to those who seek help and may be combined to create the most effective, individualized plan for treatment. Programs that offer combinations of methods have been shown to be more effective than single-method programs for smoking cessation.

According to strategies for smoking cessation outlined by clinical investigators (Wetter et al., 1998), health care professionals must begin to diagnose tobacco dependence in all smokers as a basis for intervention. AHCPR guidelines recommend that smoking be made one of the "vital signs" evaluated at each clinical visit. Techniques for assessment may include an evaluation of smoking status along with vital signs during the clinical visit. Recent investigations have noted that evaluating smoking status on a consistent basis approximately doubles the identification of smokers in health care settings and improves rates of clinician intervention (Fiore, Jorenby, & Baker, 1997). Tobacco use should be noted in the medical record, with chart reminders used to facilitate smoking status assessment (Cohen, 1984). Approximately one third of smokers who successfully quit had been advised to quit by their care provider (Fiore et al., 1997). AHCPR guidelines recommend that advice from care providers be clear, strong, and personalized. The message should include an emphasis on personal risk and the role of smoking in increasing personal risk or worsening an existing disease process. In studies in which care providers advised patients to quit, interventions raised long-term quit rates from 7.9% to 10.2% (Fiore et al., 1997). Counseling is particularly important in that, compared with younger smokers, older smokers may be less likely to believe information about the adverse health effects of smoking and more likely to consider smoking an effective coping tactic (Higgins et al., 1993). In a review of smoking cessation interventions delivered by physicians, Ockene (1987) found 1-year cessation rates from 5% to 18%.

Along with an assessment of smoking status, a smoking history is an important part of the medical database, which will guide strategies for smoking cessation (Orleans et al., 1994). Data include the number of cigarettes smoked per day and other forms of tobacco use, including chew and snuff. An evaluation of dependence on tobacco includes the presence and type of withdrawal symptoms, how soon the first cigarette of the day is smoked, and the use of cigarettes even when ill.

Clearly, an evaluation of motivation to stop smoking and commitment to the cessation process is essential. For those who are ready to quit, the development of an individualized plan for cessation—including an individual quit date, identification of specific barriers or high-risk situations for relapse, and strategies for overcoming barriers—is essential (Fiore et al., 1997). Resources may include the availability of formal smoking cessation programs or self-help and educational materials. Continued support from the health care provider is important in maintaining abstinence over time. Patients who are not yet ready to quit also may benefit from self-help and educational materials. Education should include recommendations to decrease the use of tobacco products and reinforcement of the need to quit during each patient contact.

Preventing relapse remains the primary challenge in smoking cessation programs. In patients who have sustained a myocardial infarction, 40% had resumed smoking 6 months after they had stopped, and almost 50% smoked at a 3- to 5-year follow-up (Havik & Maeland, 1988). These relapse rates are consistent with those seen in other studies, in which 30% to 50% of patients resumed smoking at 6 months. Several relapse prevention strategies have been developed (Marlatt & Gordon, 1985). Skill training to learn to identify and cope with situations in which relapse is likely to occur, identification of potentially self-defeating beliefs and expectations about smoking, and acknowledgment and acceptance of "slips" are three such interventions. Despite these and other relapse-prevention interventions, a high rate of relapse is noted in behaviorally oriented programs at 6-month follow-up (Kamarck & Lichtenstein, 1988; Kottke, Brekke, & Solberg, 1993). Fiore et al. (1997) provided guidelines designed to assist professionals in their efforts to encourage smoking cessation and prevent relapse in cessation efforts. The most important of the guidelines emphasizes adequate follow-up of the patient, particularly during the first 2 weeks of cessation, when relapse is highest (Kenford et al., 1994). Contact may include telephone calls and clinic visits focused on the development of coping strategies and reinforcement for success.

PHYSICAL ACTIVITY

An important consideration in health promotion of the older person is the initiation and maintenance of regular physical activity. The benefits of regular physical activity are well documented (Buskirk, 1985; Pate et al., 1995; Shephard, 1997) and include reduction in all-cause mortality, sudden cardiac death, and cardiovascular endpoints, such as lower incidence of acute myocardial infarction (AMI) and unfavorable lipoprotein profiles. Regular physical activity can minimize or prevent chronic problems, such as cardiovascular disease, obesity, muscle strength, osteoporosis, decreased immune function, and psychological depression (Shephard, 1997). In spite of the well-documented evidence that physical activity is beneficial, only 30% of individuals over the age of 65 report exercising regularly (Elward & Larson, 1992; Nieman, Warren, et al., 1993).

Data from the National Institute on Aging using the established population for epidemiologic studies of older people examined the association between recreational physical activity, functional status, chronic conditions, and mortality (Simonsick et al., 1993). For those elders who were classified as "high actives," mortality was reduced by one half to two thirds that of inactive elders. Individuals classified as having activity levels as "moderate to high" had decreased risk of physical impairment, rates of stroke, and risk of angina.

The role of physical activity and physical fitness in preventing and controlling coronary heart disease (CHD) is well established. Recent studies suggest that even moderate physical activity on a regular basis confers cardiopulmonary conditioning benefits (USDHHS, 1996). Regular physical activity reduces CHD risk, promotes weight loss and control, and improves musculoskeletal functioning (Paffenbarger et al., 1993). Data from several epidemiologic studies suggest that populations with habitual physical activity have decreased mortality from atherosclerotic coronary artery disease (CAD). The study by Paffenbarger, Hyde, Wing, and Hsieh (1986) of Harvard alumni showed that exercise was inversely related to cardiovascular mortality. The Framingham data showed improved cardiovascular and CHD mortality rates with increased physical activity at all ages, including older people.

Physiologic benefits of regular physical activity are related to increased high-density lipoprotein cholesterol (HDL-C) levels, reduction in blood pressure, increased cardiovascular functional capacity, decreased myocardial oxygen demand, lowered plasma insulin levels with improved glucose tolerance, and a decrease in platelet adhesiveness and fibrolytic activity. The protective effect of physical activity is seen at all ages. In patients with diagnosed CHD, preanginal exercise levels and stress tolerance are increased even with low-intensity exercise.

The physiological processes that accompany inactivity are remarkably similar to the processes of aging. These include muscle atrophy, decreased blood volume, decreased specific and nonspecific immunity, and decreased physical fitness. Specific changes in muscle composition and function have been thought to reflect the process of aging. These structural changes include a decrease in total muscle mass, decrease in number and size of type II (fast twitch) muscle fibers, loss of motor units, and decrease of the metabolic and oxidative capacity of muscle cells (Fiatarone & Evans, 1993). Essentially the same morphologic changes are seen in skeletal muscle when atrophy occurs with both disuse and aging (Fiatarone et al., 1990; Fried, Ettinger, Lind, Newman, & Gardin, 1994). Although functional decline is associated with aging, this decline can be offset with physical activity interventions (Lowenthal, Kirschner, Scarpace, Pollock, & Graves, 1994).

Benefits of Physical Activity on Cardiovascular Disease

The natural process of the aging of the cardiovascular system includes decreases in exercise cardiac output, stroke volume, maximum oxygen consumption, and heart rate (Marsiglio & Holm, 1988; Tate, Hyek, & Taffet, 1994). Although the decrease in the maximal heart rate is irreparable, the stroke volume (*SV max*) can be enhanced with regular exercise (Tate et al., 1994).

The elderly individual who engages in exercise reaps many benefits directed toward the cardiovascular system. Physical activity improves myocardial performance. Physical training of older sedentary individuals has been shown to increase peak diastolic filling of the heart and decrease the occurrence of cardiovascular diagnoses in both men and women (Levy, Cerqueira, Abrass, Schwartz, & Stratton, 1993; Posner et al., 1990). In both elderly and aged men and women, physical training has been shown to increase cardiac muscle contractility, reduce premature contractions, increase aerobic capacity, and reduce systolic blood pressure (Koro, 1990; Steinhaus et al.,

1990). In women, a strong relation exists between leisure-time physical activity and blood pressure level. Older women who are active have a 20 mmHg lower systolic blood pressure than do women who are inactive (Reaven, Barrett-Connor, & Edelstein, 1991).

The major dependent variable in research on the effectiveness of exercise training is aerobic capacity and maximum attainable heart rate. The results of research on the effectiveness of exercise training have consistently revealed improved functioning in long-term exercisers and previously sedentary adults who enroll in short-term training programs (McArdle et al., 1991). The main advantage that exercise seems to hold as a means of retaining a higher level of cardiovascular functioning is that it provides a continued stimulus for the muscle cells of the heart to undergo strong contractions so that they retain or gain contractile power.

The other advantage of exercise training is that it makes it possible for the individuals to save energy during aerobic work that is less than maximal by fulfilling the demands of the workload but placing less stress on the heart (Morey et al., 1991). Physical exercise provides strong protective benefits against every level of pathogenetic events eventuating in CAD. Blood pressure, serum lipids, blood coagulability, cardiac reserve, and the dimensions of the arteries are all directly benefited by exercise. Paffenbarger and colleagues' (1986) multidecade longitudinal study of Harvard alumni suggests that physical exercise acts prophylactically against clogged arteries. Exercise training also has favorable effects on the body's performance by increasing the efficiency of metabolism in the working muscles.

Cardiac rehabilitation following an acute cardiac event has been questioned as beneficial in elderly patients. This issue was examined in 92 ($M = 70$) elderly patients who were compared to 182 younger ($M = 54$) patients enrolled in a phase II cardiac rehabilitation program (Lavie, Milani, & Littman, 1993). For both groups, there was significant improvement in exercise capacity and reduction of obesity and unfavorable lipoproteins. The authors concluded that elderly patients should not be categorically denied the psychosocial, physical, and risk-factor benefits of secondary coronary prevention.

Benefits of Physical Activity on Weight Management

Obesity is commonly thought to be associated with increased caloric intake, but there is little evidence to support this (King & Tribble, 1991). More likely, the contributing factor to obesity includes reduced physical activity and differences in the effect of physical activity on diet-induced thermogenesis. Recent evidence suggests that physical activity is particularly important in aiding and sustaining weight loss through increased total energy expenditure, preservation of lean body mass, and changes in metabolism (King & Tribble, 1991). It is the preservation of fat-free mass (FFM, or lean tissue) that contributes to the stability of diet-induced reduction of resting metabolic rate (RMR). Some data, however, indicate that whereas FFM is preserved with exercise and diet intervention, RMR is still depressed. In spite of this, exercise induces significant reductions in fat mass (FM) as well as favorable lipoprotein changes in obese individuals (Andersen, Wadden, Bartlett, Vogt, & Weinstock, 1995; Ballor & Poehlman, 1994; Moore, Oddou, & Leklem, 1991; Racette, Schoeller, Kushner, Neil, & Herling-Iaffaldano, 1995). The exercise-induced preservation of FFM and reduction of FM explain why diet restriction and exercise may not contribute to weight loss; FFM could actually increase with exercise.

Abdominal distribution of adipose tissue is related to greater health risks than is total body fatness. Aerobic exercise promotes the loss of abdominal adipose tissue more readily than adipose tissue at other sites (Despres et al., 1984). A study examining women aged 40 to 82 years subject to 20 to 40 minutes of indoor walking four times a week demonstrated that although weight was not reduced, lean muscle mass was increased and percentage body fat was decreased (Bergman & Boyungs, 1991). Another examination used resistance training in older women with three protocols: low-intensity, high-intensity, and a control group. The high-intensity group experienced increased FFM (lean tissue), the low-intensity group experienced a decrease in FM, and both groups increased muscle strength with no change in RMR (Taaffe, Pruitt, Reim, Butterfield, & Marcus, 1993).

The fat weight gained in elderly women is often attributed to menopause; however, some data indicate that menopausal status does not appear to have an effect on obesity and body fat. Pre- and postmenopausal women were examined in a sedentary and exercise group. Nonexercisers had more body fat compared to the exercisers, regardless of menopausal status (Schaberg-Lorei, Ballard, McKeown, & Zinkgraf, 1990).

It is not only the amount of exercise but the intensity of the exercise that may be important in the mobilization of regional fat loss. In the Canadian Fitness Survey, 1,366 women and 1,257 men were measured for energy expenditure during leisure-time physical activity; maximum oxygen uptake, subcutaneous fat, and fat distribution (estimated by waist-hip ratio) also were measured. Individuals who engaged in vigorous physical activities on a regular basis had lower subcutaneous fat and waist-hip ratios than those who did not (Tremblay et al., 1991).

Progressive resistance training in both older men and older women produces a significant increase in resting energy expenditure. Following 16 weeks of strength training in healthy men (aged 50-65 years), an 8% increase in RMR was observed (Pratley et al., 1994). In a similar study with elderly men and women, a 12-week program of strength training resulted in an increased RMR as well as a significant loss of fat (Campbell, Crim, Young, Joseph, & Evans, 1995).

Benefits of Physical Activity on Lipoproteins and Glucose Tolerance

Physical activity has a beneficial reducing effect on unfavorable blood lipids and increases the HDL-C. In one study, exercise (aerobic and resistance training) added to a short-term dietary restriction program demonstrated that elderly women in the exercise group experienced reduction in low-density lipoprotein cholesterol (LDL-C), very low density lipoprotein cholesterol (VLDL-C), and triglycerides, and increases in HDL-C, compared to sedentary controls (Svendsen, Hassager, & Christiansen, 1994). Other investigations demonstrated the favorable effects of exercise on lipoproteins and glucose tolerance even without dietary restriction (Hersey et al., 1994; Seals, Hagberg, Hurley, Ehsani, & Holloszy, 1984). These same findings apply to elderly men; there are similar positive effects of either diet alone or diet plus exercise in reduction of body fat and lipoproteins (Dengel, Hagberg, Coon, Drinkwater, & Goldberg, 1994).

A comparison study (Lindheim et al., 1994) examining the effects of physical activity with and without estrogen replacement on lipids and lipoproteins in postmenopausal women was initiated with 101 sedentary women. Four randomized groups were studied: control or sedentary, exercise alone, estrogen alone, and estrogen and exercise. Systolic blood pressure was reduced in all groups; exercise alone was associated with significant decreases in total cholesterol, triglycerides, and LDL-C. Similar changes were seen with the estrogen-alone group, along with increased HDL-C.

Other studies show marked improvement in endurance following an exercise intervention, but not in lipoproteins. Thirty-two healthy sedentary women aged 67 to 85 years participated in a study examining the effects of either walking or calisthenics on lipoproteins and aerobic capacity. Following 12 weeks of 30 to 40 minutes per day exercise, the VO_2max was improved, but no changes in body weight, dietary quality, or serum lipids or lipoproteins were observed (Nieman, Henson, et al., 1993; Owens, Matthews, Wing, & Kuller, 1990).

Benefits of Physical Activity on Osteoporosis

Osteoporosis occurs as a result of both aging and menopause. A gradual decline in bone density occurs throughout middle age and is accelerated following menopause (Blair, Kohl, & Gordon, 1992). In women, estrogen is an important determinant of bone loss, and inactivity augments the loss.

The relation between physical activity and bone mineral density has been examined extensively. Bone responds to the stress of exercise and helps slow the decline in bone mineral density in older women (Haskell et al., 1992). Empirical evidence exists demonstrating less marked osteoporosis in individuals who have engaged in lifelong weight-bearing exercise and maintained adequate calcium intake (Slemenda, Miller, Hui, Reister, & Johnston, 1991). Coupling strength and weight-bearing exercise in postmenopausal women has been shown to help reduce the bone mineral density loss and increase bone density (Chow, Harrison, & Notarius, 1987; Smith, Reddan, & Smith, 1981). The increase in bone density appears even with low-intensity activity such as walking but not with other, non-weight-bearing activities such as swimming (Orwoll, Ferar, Oviatt, McClung, & Huntington, 1989).

Benefits of Physical Activity on Psychological Well-Being

Exercise contributes to psychological well-being in older people. Among women who exercised as part of a controlled intervention, those who exercised experienced improvement in perceived well-being and happiness (Moore & Bracegirdle, 1994).

Several mechanisms are thought to contribute to the association between physical activity and psychological well-being. A decrease in tyrosine hydroxylase and dihydroxyphenylalanine decarboxylase occurring with aging contributes to decreased catecholamine synthesis. An increase in monoamine oxidase activity also occurs with aging; both of these changes produce lower levels of catecholamine, which is associated with depression (Shangold, 1990).

The aging process is associated with decreased serotonin synthesis and increased serotonin metabolism; reduction of serotonin levels is associated with depression. It is well established that adults who become involved in aerobic activity experience a variety of positive effects on mood, anxiety levels, and feelings of mastery and control, leading to enhanced feelings of self-esteem (Hill, Storandt, & Malley, 1993; McAuley, Lox, & Duncan, 1993). In animal models, exercise contributes to higher levels of the catecholamine norepinephrine and serotonin, both of which prevent or relieve depression

(Brown, McCartney, & Sale, 1990). It is on this basis that exercise is used to prevent and treat depression.

Although some researchers have demonstrated positive effects of exercise on cognitive functioning (Chodzko-Zajko, 1991; Chodzko-Zajko & Moore, 1994; Stevenson & Topp, 1990), this effect is not consistently observed (Hill et al., 1993). Physical activity can sustain cerebral perfusion and cognition. A comparison of inactive retirees, physically active retirees, and elders who continued employment were examined at baseline and at a 4-year follow-up. Retirees who were physically inactive had significant declines in cerebral blood flow when compared to the physically active elders (Rogers, Schroeder, Secher, & Mitchell, 1990).

Benefits of Physical Activity on Muscle Weakness and Functional Capacity

Avoiding the decline of musculoskeletal function is particularly relevant for maintaining functional independence. The ability to modify biological decline varies across domains, but it has been suggested that the ability to delay, prevent, and reverse age-related functional losses has been highly underestimated. Deficits in activities of daily living have been linked to morbidity and mortality.

Significant and highly visible changes in body composition occur with aging. As aging occurs, there is progressive decline in FFM and increase in FM. In addition, reductions in active skeletal muscle mass occur. This loss has significant effects on bone metabolism and functional exercise capacity. The loss of muscle mass and strength, however, is not an inevitable accompaniment of aging. Instead, it is related to a decline in habitual physical activity (Shephard, 1997).

Although older individuals lose both muscle mass and muscle strength as they age, they additionally may suffer from musculoskeletal disabilities. These musculoskeletal disabilities may contribute to problems with walking and performance of activities of daily living and falls (Blair et al., 1992; Coupland, Wood, & Cooper, 1993; Gersten, 1991). A growing body of literature supports multiple benefits of physical exercise training for older adults. The effects of the loss of muscle mass can be ameliorated by physical activity directed toward muscle strength and endurance. Not only does directed physical activity improve work capacity in older people, but it improves strength and flexibility (Blumenthal et al., 1991; Buskirk, 1985; Frontera, Meredith, O'Reilly, & Evans, 1990; Frontera, Meredith, O'Reilly, Knuttgen, & Evans, 1988). Muscle mass from physical activity contributes to increased strength in older individuals and may reduce the risk of falls (Blair et al., 1992). Reports of reduced risk of fractures in both men and women are attributed to physical activity (Sorock et al., 1988).

Physical activity keeps the elderly individual from losing muscle, aerobic strength, and flexibility. A comparison of physically active and inactive elderly women ($M = 71$ years) demonstrated significant differences in endurance, walking, and flexibility as measured by the "sit and reach" test (Voorrips et al., 1993). Low-intensity aerobic exercise has been shown to improve flexibility in older people, when compared to sedentary elders (Mills, 1994). Morey et al. (1991) examined the impact of 2 years of supervised exercise in elderly veterans aged 65 to 74 on cardiovascular fitness, flexibility, and strength. Seventy-five patients exercised 3 days a week for 90 minutes, focusing on flexibility, aerobic development, and strength. After 2 years, submaximal and resting heart rates decreased, and flexibility improved, but strength did not.

Several examinations of the effects of physical activity and strength training in older people have demonstrated significant improvement in quadriceps strength, body sway, and reaction time that contribute to balance (Lord & Castell, 1994a, 1994b; Lord et al., 1993). These effects were found in groups receiving 10 and 20 weeks of a walking program and gentle exercise.

Also counteracting the picture of decline in muscle strength is evidence showing that a program of exercise can help the middle-aged and older adult compensate for the loss of muscle fibers. Muscle fibers can be strengthened and work efficiency increased through exercise training, even in persons as old as 90 years (Fiatarone et al., 1990). Inactivity can accelerate the loss of muscle strength, and the same is true of bone loss. It is possible for older individuals to benefit from exercise training, particularly if it is oriented toward promoting flexibility. Exercise can strengthen the muscles that support the joints, increase the circulation of blood to the joints, and thereby promote the repair of injured tissues and decrease the risk of injury.

Strength training interventions in older people have been demonstrated to be beneficial. A 9% to 18% increase in upper-body strength was demonstrated in healthy men and women between the ages of 70 and 79 years following 26 weeks of three times a week weight training (Hagberg et al., 1989). High-intensity strength training produces even more beneficial effects. Following dynamic high-intensity strength training, older men demonstrated a 23% increase in isometric strength for elbow flexors, a 10% increase in knee extensor strength, and a 226% increase in knee flexor strength (Frontera et al., 1988; Moritani & de Vries, 1980). In older women ($M = 69$ years), dynamic resistance training resulted in a 28% to 115% increase in upper- and lower-body strength (Charette et al., 1991). It appears that training at a sufficient intensity (10%-90% of one repetition) results in gains of muscle size and strength that mirror those achieved in young individuals (Fiatarone & Evans, 1993).

The oldest old and the frail also receive benefit from strength training. In two studies that examined the effects of strength training on the frail elderly, profound increases in strength and gait speed (48% improvement) were found, as well as a 28% increase in stair-climbing power (Fiatarone et al., 1990, 1994). Fiatarone and colleagues (1990) recruited a group of very frail 90-year-old nursing home residents to join an exercise program. At baseline, muscle size and strength balance and mobility suggested great fragility. Following only a few weeks of participation in the program, muscle size and strength had improved by as much as 174%. Walking was improved, and the tendency toward falls was reduced. In another study (Evans & Rosenberg, 1991), a 3-month exercise program resulted in doubling to tripling of muscle strength of 12 men aged 60 to 72 years.

Falls

Recently, investigators have proposed a conceptual framework that underpins the risk and sequences leading up to a fall that results in hip fracture, providing a structure both for the assessment of the risk of falls in older people and for interventions targeted toward prevention. Empirical analysis of falls and falling patterns has resulted in analysis of the interplay between fall biomechanics and bone fragility that results in fall injury. The complex interplay of events that precede a fall has been conceptualized and categorized into the following categories: the elder's neuromuscular and cognitive status, vision, and the presence of environmental hazards. These factors can initiate a fall. Second, the factors that influence the descent of the fall include the fall direction and height and muscle activity at the time of the fall. The location, impact surface, and soft tissue attenuation influence the impact of the fall. The bone mineral density and bone architecture and geometry influence the fracture occurrence. Thus, from these investigators (Meyers, Young, & Langlois, 1996), several intervention points can be identified for prevention: the appropriate assessment of physical and cognitive impairment and environmental safety, and the integrity of bone mass that is significantly influenced by nutrition and exercise.

There are a large number of clinical examinations concerning the descriptive and correlated factors that contribute to falls in older people. Investigators from the National Institute on Aging (NIA) conducted a comprehensive review of the factors. The authors categorized the risk factors into nine distinct factors associated with falls, injurious falls, and recurrent falls. General physical functioning—including impaired mobility, use of walk aides, and impaired stepping or stumbling—was the first categorical risk. Second, impaired physical activity provided a significant contribution to falls; this includes impaired activities of daily living and physical disability. Elders who engaged in vigorous physical activity were found to have a protected effect against fall risk. Gait and balance abnormalities and dizziness and vertigo constituted the third category. The measured strength of the musculoskeletal and neuromuscular system, including decreased handgrip strength, decreased joint flexion and extension, and decreased sensory discrimination were fall-related risks. Sensory difficulty, such as visual acuity and perception, was the fifth categorical risk, with demographic factors such as age and gender (women and the oldest old sustain more fall injuries) making up the sixth category. Concomitant chronic illness—such as hypotension and osteoarthritis—poor general health, and polypharmacy were categorical factors seven to eight. Last, the authors found that psychological and sociobehavioral factors contributed to fall risk (Meyers et al., 1996). These included low social interaction and activities; living alone; and impairment, either psychological, mental, or cognitive.

A number of investigations have evaluated the effects of interventions targeted toward reduction of falls. Mulrow et al. (1994) studied frail elderly residing in a nursing home who received individually tailored physical therapy three times a week for 4 months. This intervention included range of motion and exercises to enhance strength, balance, and transfer. Although no differences in range of motion, strength, or balance were achieved, the intervention group used assistive devices less frequently and were more mobile. In a study (Rubenstein et al., 1994) that included only male participants (older than 70 years), 3 months of three exercises per week were the intervention. The classes focused on lower-extremity strength training. Significant improvements were seen in the intervention group in knee and hip strength, gait, and velocity. A further intervention study by Tinetti et al. (1994), targeting more risk factors, such as medications and behavioral risk factors, demonstrated a significant difference in the number of falls between the control and intervention group.

Although there are few studies of strength training in older people, those available indicate that it is the intensity of the strength training that contributes to the strength gained (Fiatarone et al., 1994; Frontera et al., 1990; Kauffman, 1985; Thompson, Crist, Marsh, & Rosenthal, 1988). Strength training interventions for older people support increases in muscle strength that are similar in older people as in younger participants. Increases in strength range from 2.9% (Larsson, 1982) to 22% (Aniansson & Gustafsson, 1981) with low-intensity training and as high as 174% (Fiatarone et al., 1990) in sedentary elderly men and women. Significant gains in muscle size and functional mobility were observed in frail residents of nursing homes up to 96 years of age (Fiatarone et al., 1994).

Minimum Level of Physical Activity for Elders

The 1990 guidelines from the American College of Sports Medicine (ACSM) presented a position statement concerning the amount of exercise required for developing and maintaining fitness in adults, including the development of muscular strength and endurance (Haskell, 1994). This statement included a recommendation on frequency (3-5 days per week), intensity (maximum heart rate), and duration (20-60 minutes per session). Resistance training (8-12 repetitions of 8-10 different exercises) of moderate intensity was recommended for at least two times per week to maintain endurance and muscle strength. The ACSM position statement reflects the current major issue concerning physical activity in adults: There is a distinction between physical activity requirements for fitness and physical activity requirements for health.

The question remains: How much activity is necessary to achieve and maintain maximum health benefits? Examinations of the dose-response effect of physical activity have demonstrated that the most significant reductions in rates of CHD are found in individuals engaging in moderate physical activity (Haskell, 1994). The very greatest benefits occur when sedentary individuals begin a program of regular physical activity (Haskell, 1994). Thirty minutes of moderate-intensity exercise once or twice a week or 10 minutes of jogging three times a week will significantly improve aerobic capacity and body composition in previously sedentary persons (Haskell, 1994).

The Exercise Prescription

The ACSM recommendations suggest 30 minutes of exercise daily, not necessarily all at one time (Haskell, 1994). Weight-bearing is probably best for bone health, but when musculoskeletal diseases cause pain, in-water exercise is most feasible. Education on prescribing exercise is essential. Societal strategies are needed to make convenient sites for exercise available on a large scale for older persons.

Clinical Assessment

There are two major considerations when counseling older adults regarding an exercise program: the older individual's reduced maximum exercise capacity and the increased prevalence of diseases in older people that alter exercise tolerance (Hagberg, 1994).The assessment of the older adult for the purpose of evaluating or implementing an exercise plan requires consideration of the older adult's physical capacity, normal or habitual activities, and the desired outcome (see Table 4.1). Activity programs for older people must be tailored to a wide range of ages, fitness levels, and health status (Elia, 1991).

Selected high-risk patients may need to be evaluated with a physical examination and a treadmill test. Data in the history that would indicate that unsupervised exercise might be hazardous include CAD, significant valvular heart disease, cardiomyopathy, and congenital disease (Fletcher, Balady, Froelicher, Hartley, Haskell, & Pollock, 1995). Some patients may need medical intervention to control hypertension, hypercholesterolemia, or dysrhythmias prior to the initiation of an exercise program. For a small number of elderly, the risks of exercise may outweigh the potential benefits.

The debate as to the need for formal exercise testing before a patient embarks on a new program of physical activity has not been settled. However, it is generally accepted that the older person who wishes to initiate a program of high-intensity physical conditioning should have a thorough physical exam; complete blood count; biochemical test of hepatic, renal, and metabolic parameters; urinalysis; and a resting electrocardiogram (Fletcher et al., 1995; Lowenthal et al., 1994).

The goal of a physical activity/exercise program is to improve or maintain endurance, strength, and flexibility. The best criterion for cardiorespiratory fitness is maximal oxygen uptake, or aerobic power (VO_2max). The "gold standard" for this criterion is the treadmill test of VO_2max. This method is relatively expensive and requires the presence of a physician, highly trained technicians, emergency personal, and equipment. Moderate intensity activities require little need for testing maximum oxygen uptake unless the client has symptomatic heart disease or intends to undertake high-intensity exercise. Moderate-intensity activities are defined as 45% to 59% VO_2max (USDHHS, 1996).

For assessing baseline levels and quantifying improvement in endurance in older people, two "field" measures can be used. For safety and convenience, a practical walking test for the apparently healthy older adult is the Rockport Fitness Walking Test, or the 1-mile walk test (Fenstermaker,

TABLE 4.1 Evaluation of the Elderly Individual for Exercise Prescription

Goal	Rationale	Strategy
Assess risk for exercise; identify chronic disease or condition or physical limitations	Disease or physical limitations can alter the prescription	Teach self-monitoring strategies, such as heart rate; discuss safety issues; some elderly will need stress test; instruct to stop exercising if angina, bone, or joint pain occurs
Assess individual motivation factors; set realistic goals	Theory-based interventions demonstrate initiation and adherence success	Assess individual barriers to, benefits of, and support available for exercise
Evaluate dietary intake	Nutritional intake may be inadequate or imbalanced to accommodate increase in caloric expenditure	Instruct to eat diet balanced in protein, carbohydrates, and fat
Evaluate for potential injury	Injury potential with impaired balance, gait, equilibrium, orthostatic hypotension, angina, osteoarthritis	
Evaluate medications	Diuretics may predispose hypocalcemia, hypokalemia, arrhythmias, volume depletion	Review medications; consider polypharmacy; encourage adequate fluid intake with exercise
	Beta blocking agents reduce exercise tolerance	
	Insulin may require dose adjustment	
	Tranquilizers may cause orthostatic hypotension	
Include warm-up/ cool-down in prescription	Reduces potential for physical injury, postexercise hypotension, syncopy, or arrhythmias	Teach basic stretching, walking in place; teach flexibility exercises
Tailor prescription to the individual	Exercise that is enjoyable, easy to perform, convenient, and inexpensive has increased adherence	

Plowman, & Looney, 1992). For the less fit individual, the evaluator can have the individual perform an activity such as walking or stair climbing and rate the amount of perceived exertion by the Borg Perceived Exertion Scale (Borg, 1982). The Borg Perceived Exertion Scale ranges from 6 to 20. If walking for 100 feet elicits a perceived exertion rating of 12 on the Borg, then for that individual the activity is moderate in nature and would be a good indicator of fitness for the defined distance.

The exercise prescription consists of four interrelated components: intensity, frequency, duration, and mode of activity. The choice of exercise intensity or degree of energy (work) required to perform an activity is particularly important when working with older adults. The physical work capacity of the older adult is often low. Because many older adults have been sedentary for a long time, specific muscle groups are often severely deconditioned; many older adults have musculoskeletal limitations, as well. For these individuals, it is particularly important to begin with low-intensity activities (2-3 metabolic equivalents) or activities that they are comfortable performing. Adding activities of higher intensity should be done slowly when monitoring skills are established.

The frequency of the activity refers to the number of times the activity is performed. When exercise intensity levels are low, participants are encouraged to increase the frequency of the exercise, perhaps to even three or four times a day. In contrast, when in physical training or performing higher-intensity activities, the individual may be encouraged to alternate training activities with walking or cycling on every other day (Williams, 1994). Recent strategies for lifestyle exercise recommend numerous bouts of exercise throughout the day for an accumulation of energy expenditure (Gordon, Kohl, & Blair, 1993; Haskell, 1994).

Duration of an exercise period refers to the amount of time involved with the activity. By increasing the frequency and duration of a low- to moderate-intensity activity, health benefits can be realized without risking injury. Some investigators suggest that the duration of a single activity is far less important than the accumulation or volume of activities (Haskell, 1994).

The type of activity should be based on the elder's interest and resources. In selecting a form of activity for older adults, activities that are enjoyable and have a minimal potential for injury are critical. Low- to moderate-intensity activities such as walking, gardening, or cycling can be considered for an exercise program. Exercise opportunities can be incorporated into activities of daily living. Parking several blocks from the grocery store, walking to get the mail, or taking the stairs instead of the elevator are examples. Scheduled leisure time activities such as golf, swimming, and dancing are excellent activities for older adults. Water activities and use of stationary bicycles are good choices for persons with musculoskeletal limitations. Occupational or vocational activities also may provide exercise opportunities. Household activities are a source of activity. Vacuuming or cleaning can be incorporated into an exercise routine.

The few intervention studies that have been tested to increase physical activities in older adults show generally positive results. The community-based intervention Australian Heart Week resulted in a twofold increase in walking among adults over 50 years of age (Owen, Bauman, Booth, Oldenburg, & Magnus, 1995). In the Bank of America Retirees Study, a 2-year experimental study, there was a significant improvement in activity in the experimental group that received health-risk appraisal and a personalized health promotion intervention over the control groups at 2 years (Fries, Bloch, et al., 1993).

Motivational Issues and Promoting Physical Activity in Older People

Intervention in health promotion efforts targeted at the initiation and adherence to an exercise prescription in older people requires careful consideration of those factors that contribute to the increase of physical activity. Individuals need high levels of motivation to sustain an exercise program; the initial motivating factors that stimulate an individual to begin exercise may not ensure maintenance over time (McAuley & Jacobson, 1991).

Many individual models of motivation have been examined in physical activity and exercise, most notably the Theory of Reasoned Action and Social Cognitive Theory. The most salient and widely studied construct in the Social Cognitive Theory with regard to exercise behavior is Self-Efficacy. Self-efficacy cognitions are directly related to the target behavior and influence the activity chosen, the effort expended in the activity, and the persistence of the behavior (McAuley, 1993). Self-efficacy cognitions have been shown to be a significant predictor of adoption and maintenance of physical activity in community samples, treadmill exertion, home-based exercise programs, and cardiac rehabilitation programs (McAuley & Jacobson, 1991). Among older adults, self-efficacy has been explanatory in continued participation in exercise prescriptions (McAuley, 1993) and positive influence on self-esteem and perceptions of well-being in response to exercise (McAuley, Mihalko, & Bane, 1997). Self-efficacy cognitions have been shown to be predictors of long-term adherence to exercise behavior in older people (McAuley et al., 1993). Self-efficacy has been associated with physical activity, both in adoption, maintenance, adherence, and dropout (Dzewaltowski, 1994; Garcia & King, 1991; Marcus, Selby, et al., 1992).

A number of factors associated with nonadherence to physical activity programs have been identified. For example, there is evidence that an individual's social class affects physical activity patterns, in that lower socioeconomic status individuals engage in less physical activity (Ford et al., 1991). Significant empirical evidence exists that social support provides a powerful influence on health behavior, including physical activity (Sallis, Patterson, Buono, Atkins, & Nader, 1988). Social support as a specific strategy to increase physical activity and adherence has been used to prevent relapses and contribute to intergroup cohesiveness and intergroup competition (King et al., 1988).

Barriers to exercise may be salient in contributing to exercise behavior. Barriers to physical activity may include time, effort, and obstacles. Barriers may include lack of knowledge, skills, and social support, as well as cost and family obligations (Sallis & Hovell, 1990).

NUTRITIONAL MANAGEMENT

Energy Requirements

Energy requirements have been noted to decrease with age. The mechanism proposed is a decrease in resting energy expenditure related to declines in muscle mass and level of physical activity (Lipschitz, 1995). Nutritional recommendations have included a decrease in average energy intake of 600 kcal/day for men and 300 for women (Food and Nutrition Board, 1989). However, the current recommended dietary allowances (RDAs) do not address the needs of persons over age 51 and do not acknowledge that older adults have unique nutritional needs (Food and Nutrition Board, 1989).

Although these preliminary results may have implications for health promotion in older people, diets that contain less than 1,800 kcal/day may provide inadequate amounts of essential nutrients, including calcium, iron, and vitamins needed for good health. Decreased metabolic rate and reduced levels of physical activity in older people result in reduced caloric need and often in decreased intake. This reduction in intake also may result in a decreased consumption of essential nutrients. Interventions designed to support the nutritional needs of older people must focus on the intake of nutrient-rich foods, including adequate intake of protein, vitamins, and minerals (Rudman & Cohan, 1991).

Nutritional Assessment

Nutritional status in older people reflects the degree to which physiologic requirements for essential nutrients are being met. The nutritional assessment evaluates dietary and other nutrition-related indicators to determine the need for clinical intervention. Although nutritional status of older people may be, for the most part, satisfactory, routine screening of nutritional status may detect nutritional deficiency or potential overload in the preclinical stage so that nutritional support and counseling can be initiated to improve dietary intake. The assessment process consists of two phases: screening for risk identification and assessment, to establish relevant goals and strategies for facilitating nutrient intake.

The goals of the screening process are to identify elderly who may be at nutritional risk or who require ongoing assessment (DeHoog, 1996). Elderly individuals may be at risk for inadequate nutrition for a number of reasons. Individual, economic, environmental, or cultural factors may include a lack of education regarding appropriate nutrition, financial limitations, physical disabilities that restrict food purchase and preparation, or social isolation (McCormack, 1997). Awareness of the potential for nutritional deficit is also important in patients who have a primary diagnosis associated with malnutrition, such as alcoholism; alteration in cognitive function; chronic myocardial, renal, or pulmonary insufficiency; malabsorption syndromes; history of recent surgery, particularly surgery of the gastrointestinal tract; and multiple medication use (Ham, 1994).

Clinical decision making should focus on the history of or evidence of anorexia, early satiety, changes in taste and smell, nausea, change in bowel habits, fatigue, or memory loss. A progressive decline in sensory acuity associated with aging may have a negative impact on the enjoyment of eating and lead to reduced dietary intake (Horwath, 1991). Physical findings that also may provide clues to the presence of nutritional deficits include poor dentition, ill-fitting dentures, angular stomatitis, and glossitis, which is common in a number of vitamin deficiencies. Pressure ulcers or poorly healing wounds, edema, dehydration, and poor dental status are common physical manifestations of nutritional inadequacies.

Cultural and psychosocial factors are also important to evaluate when assessing dietary status. Limited income has been linked with reduced access to nutrient-dense foods as well as inadequate facilities for food storage and food preparation (Ham, 1992). Social isolation also must be considered. Factors such as lack of transportation, living alone, or loss of functional ability may negatively affect dietary intake. Factors such as adequate income to purchase food, adequacy of food preparation facilities, access to shopping areas, and social context are essential to sufficient intake. Opportunities for social interaction with others, including increased physical activity, may have a positive impact on well-being and food intake (Horwath, 1991). Cultural and religious practices may determine the types of foods acceptable and are particularly important to consider when developing dietary interventions.

The nutritional assessment quantifies nutritional risk through evaluation of individual nutritional history; physiologic data, including anthropometric measures of height, weight, and weight patterns; and lab values indicative of nutritional deficit. A diet history is essential to obtain needed information on usual patterns of food intake and food selection (DeHoog, 1996). The overall goal of the diet history is to evaluate the quality and adequacy of nutrient content for each individual. Dietary intake may be evaluated either by assessment of retrospective intake data or through a summary of prospective intake data. Methods for obtaining dietary intake include 24-hour recall, food frequency questionnaires, food records, and direct observation of food intake. The 24-hour recall method requires remembering food consumption from the previous day. The food frequency questionnaire requires remembering the number of times per day, week, or month that particular foods are eaten. Both of these recall methods are sometimes used together to obtain a more comprehensive assessment of dietary intake. The food record involves recording all dietary intake for at least 3 days, including 2 weekdays and 1 weekend day. These data are then assessed to obtain an average daily intake evaluation. Observational methods are best suited to a clinical setting and involve observation and recording of actual food intake as well as an evaluation of the social context and use of assistive techniques. Dietary intake is evaluated by the dietary guidelines and food guide pyramid or by RDAs.

Clinical Examination

The clinical examination includes the physical examination and an associated medical history. Physical signs of nutritional deficiency are often manifest in the skin, hair, teeth, tongue, and mucous membranes. Significant findings on examination that indicate nutritional deficit include muscle wasting and weakness; and skin condition, including pallor, dermatitis, wounds that do not heal, bruising, and hydration. Mucous membranes are assessed for integrity, hydration, and bleeding (DeHoog, 1996). Physical signs and symptoms require confirmation with a dietary evaluation and assessment of laboratory data.

Biochemical Assessment

Biochemical assessment of nutritional status is an objective measure that can be evaluated in conjunction with clinical and anthropometric data. The use of serial lab tests may be more accurate than a single test and allows evaluation of trends in nutritional status over time and long-term nutrient intake (DeHoog, 1996). As part of a comprehensive evaluation, biochemical and hematological findings are more sensitive indicators of nutritional status than observable signs and symptoms. Hemoglobin, hematocrit, complete blood count with differential, serum albumin, total protein, serum glucose, and urinalysis have been recommended.

Anthropometric Data

Anthropometric measurement includes height, weight, body mass index, skinfolds thickness, and circumference measurements. These measurements provide estimates of body weight and fat for determining nutritional status. A gradual increase in weight has been noted with advancing age, peaking in the early 40s in men and in the 50s in women. However, after age 70, many individuals experience a reduction in weight, with body fat constituting a greater percentage of total weight compared with those of younger age. Fat distribution also has been shown to change with age. Truncal and intra-abdominal fat consistently increase, and limb fat diminishes.

Skinfold measurements are often employed to estimate fat and muscle stores. Skinfold measures provide an indication of body density and require precise skinfolds calipers designed to apply constant pressure throughout their range of motion (Keller & Thomas, 1995). Although the triceps skinfold is the most frequently obtained, multiple skinfolds are much more reliable than single measurements. The skinfold technique as a measurement of body fatness is based on two assumptions: (a) that the thickness of the subcutaneous adipose tissue reflects a constant proportion of the total body fat, and (b) that the sites selected for measurement represent the average thickness of the subcutaneous adipose tissue (Keller & Thomas, 1995; Lukaski, 1987).

Anthropometric measures vary with age and gender equations. Body density differences between men and women can be attributed to differences in fat distribution, internal to external fat ratio, and gender-specific essential fat (Pollock & Jackson, 1984). In older people, subscapular and supra iliac skinfolds are the best predictors of fat stores in men, whereas the triceps skinfolds and thigh measurements are of greater value in women. In extreme age groups, the proportion of body water in lean tissue varies considerably and may affect the density of the FFM and, thus, the accuracy of equations predicting body density (Pollock & Jackson, 1984). Total body water also is decreased in parallel to declines in lean body mass. Evaluating ideal body weight for height can be employed to determine if a patient is underweight. Tables are available for older persons that provide a guide to their ideal body weight. These are based on an assessment of height, weight, and body frame. On the basis of these tables, being significantly underweight is defined as being 15% below the ideal weight for that individual patient. However, current tables are based on relatively small samples and often are not representative of the individual being evaluated.

A more convenient assessment is the determination of the Body Mass Index (BMI). The BMI is an expression of relative weight, in this case, body weight relative to height. BMI is calculated as weight (in kilograms) divided by the square of height (m^2). Use of BMI is limited for reflecting body fat because it does not distinguish fat weight from nonfat weight (Keller & Thomas, 1995). Thus, BMI reflects relative weight of both lean tissue and fat tissue (Lohman, 1992). It is generally recommended that persons over the age of 65 have a BMI between 24 and 29. The BMI, however, does not reflect the percentage of body fat and may be increased in those with higher lean body mass. Using this measure, obesity has been defined as a BMI 27.3 kg/m^2 in women and 27.8 kg/m^2 in men (Keller & Thomas, 1995), which corresponds to approximately 20% above the ideal body weight according to Metropolitan Life Insurance Company tables. Individuals with a high BMI should be further examined for relative fatness, fat distribution, or both. Because of the low sensitivity of this measure, BMI should be viewed as a screening device and the results interpreted with caution.

Although adiposity may be measured more directly, using skinfold thickness or bioelectric impedance, these techniques are not necessary to identify obesity. More recently, increased attention has been given to measures of central fat distribution, particularly the ratio of waist circumference to hip circumference (Keller & Thomas, 1995). Waist-to-hip ratio (WHR) is the simplest method for determining regional fat, providing information on the anatomical distribution of adipose tissue on the waist and hips. The waist circumference is measured at the narrowest spot between the ribs and hips, or, when a narrow point is not evident, the midpoint between the lowest rib and the iliac crest. The hip circumference is measured at the widest circumference over the great trochanter. The WHR is calculated by dividing the waist measurement by the hip measurement (Keller & Thomas, 1995). A WHR greater than 1.0 in men and 0.9 in women is associated with substantial increase in risk for hypertension, stroke, and diabetes (Bray, 1987). Waist-hip ratio correlates directly with blood pressure, blood glucose levels, glucose-stimulated insulin levels, and triglyceride levels, and inversely with HDL levels. In prospective studies, a high waist-hip ratio is an independent predictor of non-insulin-dependent diabetes mellitis (Ohlson et al., 1985) and cardiovascular morbidity and mortality (Lapidus, Bengtsson, & Lissner, 1990), even after adjusting for BMI.

Although waist-hip ratios are correlated with visceral fat, independent associations of WHR and visceral fat are not always significant. A "conicity" index, which assumes that a body shape changes from a cylinder to double cone when fat is accumulated in and around the abdomen, is almost independent of body fatness, as it includes weight, height, and waist circumference (Valdez, Seidell, Ahn, & Weiss, 1993; van der Kooy & Seidell, 1993).

Overnutrition

Although obesity in older people has been associated with a shortened life expectancy, the degree of obesity related to morbidity and mortality is not well understood. Hypertension, diabetes, and degenerative arthritis compose the central triad that frequently accompanies obesity, each of which threatens length and quality of life. Overconsumption of calories, particularly as fat, and declining levels of physical activity have made obesity a major public health problem in the United States. One of the stated hallmarks of aging is an increasingly higher percentage of body fat. This percentage is a function of the reciprocal decline in lean body mass along with an absolute increase in body fat, both of which are sensitive to the effect of physical exercise.

Obesity is a condition characterized by an excessive storage of energy in the form of body fat, and it is identified when a person is more than 20% over ideal body weight (McArdle et al., 1991). *Overweight* is defined as excess body weight usually greater than 10% above ideal weight. The preferred method of determining obesity is by estimating the percentage of body weight that is fat. The term obesity is applied to men whose body fat is more than 20% of body weight and to women whose body fat is more than 30% of body weight (McArdle et al., 1991). Approximately 20% of participants over the age of 65 are significantly overweight. Obesity results from an imbalance between caloric intake and energy expenditure. This imbalance may be due to a number of factors, including inactivity, reduced metabolic rate, or reduced mobility.

It is clear that weight reduction can ameliorate many of the adverse effects of obesity. Significant decreases in serum glucose levels have been reported within days of beginning calorie-restricted diets, and hypoglycemic agents frequently can be decreased or eliminated (Pi-Sunyer, 1993). Similarly, weight loss is associated with significant reductions in blood pressure and lipid levels. Decreases in systolic blood pressure of 10 to 18 mmHg and in diastolic blood pressure of 9 to 13 mmHg have been reported with weight loss of 8 to 10 kg (Tuck, Sowers, & Dornfeld, 1981). Results from a meta-analysis of 70 studies of the effects of weight loss on lipid profile indicate that for every kilogram decrease in body weight, LDL-C falls by 0.77 mg/dl, and total cholesterol falls by 1.93 mg/dl; once weight has stabilized, HDL-C increases by 0.35 mg/dl per kilogram lost (Dattilo & Kris-Etherton, 1992). Consistent with these findings, weight reduction over time among the Framingham population was associated with decreased risks of CHD (Ashley & Kannel, 1974).

Undernutrition

Weight loss is perhaps the most important finding indicating the presence of malnutrition. Recent studies have indicated that this finding in patients with serious disease is a poor prognostic sign and is associated with increased morbidity and mortality (Sullivan, Walls, & Lipschitz, 1991). To be significant, weight loss must be involuntary. Weight loss must have exceeded 10% or more of body weight in 6 months, 7.5% or more in 3 months, or 5% or more in 1 month. In older persons, any weight loss that clearly cannot be ascribed to alterations in fluid balance should be taken seriously. It must be emphasized that significant malnutrition can be present in individuals who are not underweight. Any significant weight loss that is involuntary indicates that nutritional intake is inadequate and that the individual's needs are not being met. Additional clinical evidence for undernutrition includes midarm circumference and skinfolds thickness less than the 10th percentile and serum albumin less than 3.5 gm/dl (Ham, 1992). Additional objective measures include reduced serum hemoglobin and transferrin levels (Silver & Morley, 1993).

There is evidence that indicates that malnutrition is highly significant in older persons. Being underweight or losing weight is associated with increased morbidity and mortality in older persons. There is even suggestive evidence that voluntary weight loss may be associated with an increased adverse outcome in older persons. To determine if the patient is underweight or has lost weight requires an evaluation of body composition (Nutrition Screening Initiative, 1994). In this regard, virtually every anthropometric measure of body composition employs height as the reference point. In both men and women, height decreases by approximately 1 cm per decade after the age of 20. This is

caused by vertebral bone loss, increased laxity of vertebral supportive liga-
ments, reductions in disk spaces, and alterations in posture. Historical esti-
mations of height are frequently inaccurate in older people, and its measurement is difficult in patients with significant postural abnormalities. For this
reason, it has been suggested that alternatives to height should be used in the
development of standards for body composition for older people. Options
suggested include arm length and knee-height measurements.

The initial approach to management should be a careful attempt to identify
the cause of the weight loss and, if found, to aggressively attempt correction.
Identifying a potentially treatable cause such as drug use (digoxin,
fluoxytene), thyrotoxicosis, and depression usually can result in weight gain
if the underlying condition is corrected with appropriate medical interventions. Other conditions that may well contribute to weight loss that are potentially improvable include social or economic isolation, difficulties with cooking or feeding as a consequence of physical disability, dental or swallowing
problems, and not providing palatable or preferred foods. Failure to identify a
cause for weight loss is generally accompanied by a poor prognosis despite
aggressive medical and nutritional interventions.

Nutritional needs and care of elderly persons are directed toward meeting
their physiologic and psychological needs (McCormack, 1997). These needs
change depending on the aging process, chronic and acute disease, use of
medication, and the emotional and mental state of the individual.

Older persons who have experienced weight loss are consuming inadequate calories to meet their needs. The nutritional aim must be to increase caloric intake, with interventions focused on specific causative factors. Interventions designed to improve access to nutrient-rich foods and increase oral
intake include provision of foods in an acceptable form and environment, use
of home delivery meals where appropriate, and use of nutritional supplements.

Increasing dietary intake can be achieved by assuring the use of food that
is nutritious and pleasant to eat. Four or five smaller meals per day are often
more acceptable than three large meals. Meals high in both protein and fats
should be encouraged, using nutritional supplements that are calorie-dense
and high in protein. Improvements in serum albumin, total lymphocyte count,
serum cholesterol, and hemoglobin have been noted when liquid nutritional
supplements have been given to elderly nursing home patients. Providing
supplements with meals is not recommended, as total caloric intake will
not be improved. Nutritional supplements also may be used between meals
to prevent weight loss in older people. If shopping or meal preparation is
a problem, alternatives such as community resources, nutrition programs,
and home-delivered meals should be investigated. Community nutrition pro-

grams exist in many communities and provide social stimulation along with hot, nutritional meals. Transportation services for grocery shopping or assistance with shopping needs also may be available in the community. Home-delivered meal programs such as "Meals on Wheels" may be available to provide at least one hot meal per day.

Protein Requirements

The current RDA for protein is 0.8 grams per kilogram of body weight for younger and middle-aged people. Recent findings indicate that this figure may be insufficient for older adults because the amount of lean body mass diminishes, particularly in regard to frailty (Evans & Rosenberg, 1991). The protein intake of older people should not be lower than that of younger adults, and older people may require more dietary protein per unit of body weight to maintain nitrogen equilibrium at the customary level of energy intake (Young, Munro, & Fukayama, 1989). Studies in older people have shown that, even in healthy elderly participants, the requirements for protein are increased (Gersovitz, Motil, Munro, Scrimshaw, & Young, 1982). A protein intake of 1 g/kg body weight is recommended in healthy elderly to maintain nitrogen balance (Campbell et al., 1995). However, more research is needed, because protein intake is particularly important for older people, especially those with low body weight.

Protein deficiency is rare in the healthy elderly population (Munro, Suter, & Russell, 1987). However, protein-calorie undernutrition may be a problem for some elderly, particularly those who live alone. Protein deficiencies contribute to edema, chronic eczema, fatigue, muscle weakness, and tissue wasting. Wound healing is impaired, and immune response may be negatively affected. The presence of acute or chronic diseases further increases protein requirements. Adequate protein intake is particularly important in wound healing, in which inadequate protein intake adversely affects outcome.

Dietary Carbohydrate Intake

As with younger people, carbohydrates constitute the most abundant source of calories for older people. A diversity of carbohydrates is essential to health in older people. Grains, vegetables, and fruits are superior sources of carbohydrate because they supply not only calories but other necessary nutrients, minerals, and vitamins. Carbohydrates supply most of the fiber content of the diet, which is critical in older people who are prone to forms of immobility and altered gastrointestinal motility.

A reduced glucose tolerance renders older people more susceptible to temporary hypoglycemia or hyperglycemia. According to Reaven (1995), approximately one quarter of the nondiabetic population experiences alterations in glucose tolerance. Compensatory mechanisms include secretion of excess amounts of insulin, which may be associated with the development of a number of physiologic abnormalities, including glucose intolerance, hypertension, elevated serum triglycerides, and reduced HDL-C.

Insulin sensitivity may be improved by reducing the use of sugar and increasing the amount of complex carbohydrate and soluble fiber in the diet. There is no RDA for carbohydrate, although most diets contain 45% to 50% of calories as carbohydrate. Current recommendations favor an increase in complex carbohydrate to at least 55% of calories, which improves intake of vitamins, minerals, and fiber.

Dietary Fat Intake

Aging does not alter requirements for essential lipids. However, the Committee on Diet and Health of the Food and Nutrition Board (1989) recommended that fat calories should represent no more than 30% of total daily calories, with less than 10% supplied by saturated fat (USDHHS, 1988). The restriction on dietary fat is derived largely from the causative role that dietary fat, particularly saturated fat, plays in the promotion of high cholesterol levels and CAD. Serum cholesterol levels in men tend to peak during middle age and drop slightly, whereas cholesterol levels in women continue to rise with age. Reducing total dietary fat, especially in the amount of saturated fat and cholesterol in the diet, can lower blood cholesterol levels and subsequent risk of heart disease. Although there is no direct available evidence that dietary changes can reduce risk of cardiovascular disease in older people, there is no reason to believe that the same environmental factors leading to decreased risk in the younger population will not continue to be effective in later years. People should limit dietary fat, especially fat found in meat and dairy products, to no more than 30% of total kilocalories; this also supports principles of weight control and cancer prevention.

Dietary Cholesterol Intake

Serum cholesterol values do tend to fall with advancing age, but coronary artery death rates continue to rise (National Institutes of Health [NIH] Consensus Development Conference Statement, 1993). Atherosclerosis represents a dynamic process in which cholesterol plays a role. For patients with borderline or elevated cholesterol levels, the National Cholesterol Education Program (NCEP; 1996) recommended that primary care providers instruct patients in the use of a cholesterol-lowering diet. The Step I diet recommended by the NCEP has less than 300 mg per day of cholesterol and 8% to 10% of total calories from saturated fatty acids. For patients who fail to adequately reduce their cholesterol levels on this diet, the Step II diet is recommended, which has less than 200 mg per day of cholesterol and less than 7% of total calories from saturated fatty acids. The NCEP provides guidelines for foods to choose or decrease for the Step I or Step II diets. The value of serum or HDL-C in the prediction of CAD is less clear for older people than it is for younger participants. Thus, the efficacy of aggressive dietary or pharmacological attempts to lower cholesterol in those over age 70 has not been substantiated.

Dietary Fiber Intake

Dietary fiber refers to primarily indigestible, nonstarch polysaccharides that are components of many foods from plant sources. Dietary fiber has been classified in two categories based on its solubility in water. The water-soluble fibers are found primarily in oat bran, fresh fruits, and beans. Water-insoluble fibers are found primarily in wheat bran and in vegetables including carrots and broccoli.

Water-soluble dietary fiber has been found to significantly lower elevated serum cholesterol levels. Although the mechanism is unclear, it is thought that fiber binds bile acids and slows the rate of lipid absorption (Council on Scientific Affairs, 1989). This hypocholesterolemic action is a function of a number of related factors, including the amount of water-soluble fiber consumed and initial serum lipid levels. Neither serum triglycerides nor HDL-C levels have been shown to be affected by dietary fiber intake.

Although data remain inconclusive, population studies suggest a relation between a high dietary fiber intake and protection against cardiovascular disease, diabetes, and obesity. Use of oat bran in association with an overall lowered fat intake has been recommended as a cost-effective intervention in the treatment of hypercholesterolemia (Kinosian & Eisenberg, 1988). Clinical intervention trials that have examined the effect of oat bran intake on cholesterol levels have reported a decrease in total serum cholesterol of approximately 10% in participants with elevated cholesterol levels (Ripsin et al., 1992). Recommended nutrient intakes are presented in Table 4.2.

TABLE 4.2 Nutrient Requirements for Older People

Nutrient	Recommended Dietary Allowance	Maximum	Alteration Manifested in Signs/Symptoms	Reference
Protein	0.8-1.0 gr/kg	1.5-2.0 g/kg	Decrease: edema, chronic eczema, fatigue, muscle weakness, tissue wasting, impaired wound healing, negative immune response	Campbell, Crim, Dallal, Young, & Evans (1994); Carter (1991); Evans & Rosenberg (1991); Fukagawa & Young (1987); Gersovitz, Motil, Munro, Scrimshaw, & Young (1982); Opper & Burakoff (1994); Young, Munro, & Fukayama (1989)
Carbohydrate	55%-60% of total calories	Increase in complex carbohydrate to at least 55% of calories	Decrease: reduced caloric intake; deficit in nutrient, mineral, and vitamin intake; complications associated with decreased intake of fiber; altered gastrointestinal motility or gastrointestinal immobility; insulin sensitivity	Carter (1991)

Fat	See next cell	< 30% of total daily calories; < 10% from saturated fat	Excess: risk of coronary artery disease	U.S. Department of Health and Human Services (1988)
Cholesterol	See next cell	Step 1 Diet: < 300 mg/day, of which 8%-10% of total calories come from saturated fatty acids	Excess: atherosclerosis	National Cholesterol Education Program (1996)
		Step II Diet: < 200 mg/day, of which < 7% of total calories come from saturated fatty acids		National Cholesterol Education Program (1996)
Fiber	See next cell	25-35 g/day	Decrease: elevated serum cholesterol levels, higher rate of lipid absorption, less protection against cardiovascular disease, diabetes, and obesity	Council on Scientific Affairs (1989); Kinosian & Eisenberg (1988); Ripsin et al. (1992)

Alcohol Intake

Moderate alcohol intake is thought to confer some beneficial cardiovascular effects that include increases in HDL and anti-platelet effects. Data seem to indicate that intake of red wine provides stronger cardioprotective effects compared with other alcoholic beverages, suggesting that factors in addition to the alcohol itself may exert protective benefits (Renaud & de Lorgeril, 1992). Efforts to understand the significantly reduced mortality rates from CHD in France have implicated the antioxidant actions of phenolic in red wine.

Vitamin Requirements

Studies have shown that dietary intake of many vitamins is inadequate in older people. For some nutrients, higher RDAs may need to be developed for the "oldest of the old" in this country (McCormack, 1997). Deficiencies of vitamins and trace elements are observed in almost one third of all elderly (Chandra, 1997). Surveys indicate that a large percentage of elderly people consume less than two thirds of the RDA of vitamins. Vitamins A and D, as well as several B vitamins, are frequently deficient in the diets of older adults. Vitamin inadequacy may be related to poverty and social isolation, both of which are relevant to the elderly population.

The health benefit of supplementing the daily diet with certain vitamins that demonstrate antioxidant properties has been widely studied for the effects that these vitamins can exert at the cellular level. The biophysiological processes of aerobic metabolism generate certain unstable biochemical by-products, known as "free radicals." The majority of free radicals that affect cellular health are oxygen compounds. These molecules can have toxic effects on body tissue by causing damage to biological macromolecules such as DNA, carbohydrates, and proteins (Stahl & Sies, 1997). The process, termed *oxidation,* has been associated with the pathological processes of various diseases, such as diabetes, cancer, and CHD.

Most of the body's cholesterol is shuttled through the blood inside carriers known as low-density lipoproteins, or LDLs. LDL is harmful only if it becomes oxidized through any of the numerous chemical reactions involving potent molecular fragments known as free radicals. Once oxidized, LDLs can be transformed into the raw ingredients of plaque, thus contributing to the atherosclerotic process (Stahl & Sies, 1997).

Antioxidant defense systems exist at the intracellular level. Their first function is to "scavenge," that is, to decompose or neutralize free radical substances. Cellular antioxidants fall into three classes: endogenously synthesized compounds with antioxidant activity, such as uric acid; exogenously derived antioxidant nutrients, such as the tocopherols (vitamin E), ascorbic acid (vitamin C), and beta carotene (a vitamin A precursor); and nonnutrient antioxidants such as bioflavonoids and polyphenols (Dreosti, 1996).

Vitamin C. Vitamin C is one of the most powerful natural antioxidants and is also a pro-oxidant. It exerts its mechanism of action primarily as a scavenger of free radicals and nonradical compounds such as hydrogen peroxide, which act in a similar manner in biological systems (Stahl & Sies, 1997). Vitamin C prevents the oxidation of LDL-C and preserves vitamin E and beta carotene levels during oxidative stress. The major food sources of vitamin C are fruits, especially citrus, kiwi, and cherries; melons; and vegetables such as green leafy vegetables, tomatoes, broccoli, and cabbage. The minimum dosage found to be effective in comparative studies is 50 mg per day, obtained either through diet or through supplements (Enstrom, Kanim, & Klein, 1992). Although some data hypothesize increases in urinary oxalate concentrations with high intakes of vitamin C, other studies found a decrease in oxalate renal stones with high (> 1,500 mg) doses (Hathcock, 1997).

The effectiveness of ascorbic acid in the prevention of CHD is hypothesized, and three possible mechanisms of action have been proposed. Ascorbic acid may retard the development of atherosclerosis by affecting the integrity of the arterial wall and aid in the biosyntheses of collagen. It may alter the metabolism of cholesterol by mediating the conversion of cholesterol to bile acids, a transformation that is dependent on the action of vitamin C. Finally, it may have an effect on triglyceride levels through modulation of lipoprotein lipase activity (Lynch, Gaziano, & Frei, 1996). Numerous in vitro studies also have suggested another mode of action, that is, the prevention of atherogenic, oxidative modification of LDL-C (Lynch et al., 1996). Specific functions of vitamin C include the protection of polyunsaturated fatty acids (PUFAs) against auto-oxidation and protection against oxidative damage at the cellular level by modulation of the immune response and by decreasing the propensity of platelets to adhere to the vessel wall (Lynch et al., 1996). Two major epidemiological studies (the Health Professionals Study and the Nurses Study) have not demonstrated any reduction in acute cardiac events related to vitamin C use (Stampfer et al., 1993).

Vitamin C is an antioxidant on its own, as well as for the "repairs" of other radicals such as vitamin E (Gey, 1998). The hydrophilic vitamin C can recycle the vitamin E radical (the major chain-breaking antioxidant in the lipid phase). There is a need, however, for an appropriate vitamin C to E ratio. Moderate to excessive vitamin E supplements of 70 to 1,050 mg substantially lower plasma vitamin C in a dose-dependent manner and produce a direct decrease in the resistance of erythrocytes to H_2O_2 perioxidation (Gey, 1998). There is a pro-oxidative property of vitamin E (> 70 mg in smokers, > 140 mg in nonsmokers) if not accompanied by sufficient increases in vitamin C (Gey, 1998). A molar vitamin C-vitamin E ratio of more than 0.6 to 0.8 is associated with increased risk of CHD, whereas ratios of more than 1.3 to 1.5 mg may be desirable (Gey, 1998).

Studies have indicated inadequate dietary intake of vitamin C in older people. There is no evidence, however, that vitamin C deficiency is of any clinical relevance in healthy elderly or that replacement with megadoses of vitamin C is of any clinical value. In elderly participants with chronic debilitating diseases, there is some evidence that vitamin C supplementation improves the rate of wound and pressure ulcer healing. There is little evidence that megadoses (71,000 mg/day) of vitamin C have any relevant side effects, although falsely negative occult bloods have been reported, as have inaccuracies in serum and urine glucose determinations. Vitamin C deficiency may present with symptoms of lassitude and fatigue. Purpura, capillary hemorrhaging, bleeding from the gums, and delayed wound healing are frequent complaints of older people. Encouraging the consumption of vitamin C-rich foods may be the most effective way of improving vitamin C nutriture of older people. Vitamin C also may have a role in cataract prevention. The current RDA is 60 mg for both men and women over age 51 years, with an increase to 100 mg/day in cigarette smokers.

Thiamine. Clinically relevant deficiencies of the B vitamins are very rare in older people. Thiamine deficiency, however, is common in elderly alcoholics and can be an important contributing factor in the development of disordered cognition, neuropathies, and perhaps cardiomyopathies.

Folate Acid. Like thiamine, folate deficiency in older people is predominantly found in alcoholics. It is also common in elderly participants who are taking drugs that interfere with folate metabolism (trimethoprim, methotrexate, and Dilantin) or in disorders associated with increased folate needs, such as hemolytic anemia and ineffective erythropoiesis. Folate deficiency may result in cognitive loss or significant depression and should always be evaluated in the work-up of elderly participants with a memory disorder.

Vitamin B12. Low serum vitamin B12 concentrations have been shown to occur in as many as 10% of otherwise healthy elderly participants. Recent research suggests that sufficient levels of B12 play a vital role in the health of elderly persons, and adequate intake may prevent decline in cognitive function associated with aging (Rosenberg & Miller, 1992). Many comprehensive work-ups indicate early pernicious anemia, the most common cause of vitamin B12 deficiency, whereas in others no obvious cause can be identified. B12 deficiency classically causes a severe megaloblastic anemia. Additional manifestations of B12 deficiency can include gait disorders, sensory and motor neurologic deficits, and memory loss. Low B12 blood levels are closely linked with a poor response by the body's natural defense system. Among those over age 65, B12 deficiency has been linked to a less effective immune response (Chandra, 1990). However, further studies are needed to see if B12 supplements can improve the immune response in individuals with low blood levels of the vitamin.

This vitamin should be measured routinely in the work-up of any elderly individual with disordered cognition or depression, and replacement therapy should be given to any individual in whom low serum levels are found. A value below 150 pg/mL is suspect and should result in the commencement of replacement therapy. The usual cause of vitamin B12 deficiency is a loss of gastric intrinsic factor, although elderly people with hypochlorhydria or achlorhydria may also malabsorb cobalamin, leading to pernicious anemia. Those with either of these conditions may require a higher dietary vitamin B12 intake than is presently recommended. Recent research has shown that increased serum levels of vitamins B6, B12, and folate confer protection against elevated homocysteine, an independent risk factor for cardiovascular disease, depression, and certain neurologic deficits (Selhub, Jacques, Wilson, Rush, & Rosenberg, 1993; Stampfer et al., 1992). For many elderly persons, nutritional status for these nutrients is less than optimal and should receive special attention.

Homocystinemia. Homocysteinemia is an inborn error of metabolism characterized by vascular abnormalities and frequent arterial and venous thrombosis. According to D'Angelo and Selhub (1997), there are three specific causes: (a) deficiency of cystathionine synthase, a pyridoxal phosphate-dependent enzyme (vitamin B6); (b) deficiency of methyltetra-hyofolate homocysteine methyl transferase, a cobalamin-dependent enzyme (vitamin B12); and (c) deficiency of methylenetetrahydrofolate reductase, a folate-dependent enzyme (vitamin B complex). Homocysteine damages cultured endothelial cells and stimulates growth of cultured smooth muscle by increased formation of cyclin messenger RNA. The thrombolic effects of homocysteine have been attributed to its effects on multiple coagulation factors, including platelets, tissue factor, activated protein C, thrombovane, lipoprotein(a) binding to fibrin, and factors V, VII, and XII (D'Angelo & Selhub, 1997). Many individuals with cardiovascular, cerebrovascular disease have elevated homocysteine levels (Boushey, Beresford, Omenn, & Motulsky, 1995). Moderate hyperhomocystienemia is a significant and independent risk factor for arteriosclerosis, comparable to the risk of smoking, hypertension, and hypercholesterolemia. In the Framingham cohort, participants with deficiencies in folate, vitamin B6, and B12 had elevated levels of homocysteine (Selhub et al., 1993). These data were similar to that of the Nurses Health Study (80,082 nurses), in which those with the highest intakes of folate and vitamin B6 had substantially reduced risk of CHD (Verhoef, Stampfer, & Rimm, 1998). The lowest risk was among women with intakes of folate of more than 400 micromg per day and vitamin B6 of more than 3 mg per day.

Subclinical deficiencies of one or more of the B vitamins, B6, B12, and folate may lead to homocysteinemia because they are cofactors for enzymes involved in homocysteine metabolism. Inadequate plasma levels of one or more of these vitamins may contribute to a majority of the cases of elevated homocysteine in older people (Selhub et al., 1993), and supplementing the diet with these vitamins is recommended for this age group (Stampfer et al., 1993). According to recent data from healthy men (Jacob, Wu, Henning, & Swendseid, 1994), the current recommended dietary allowance for folate for adult men may not adequately protect against homocysteinemia. The addition of 1 mg of vitamin B12 to dietary supplements containing folic acid has been recommended (Morrison, Schaubel, Desmeules, & Wigle, 1996).

Although it has been recognized that high levels of plasma homocysteine may cause occlusive vascular disease, it has been found that elevations of this amino acid are associated with increased risk of atherosclerosis (Clark et al., 1991). Three concerns about the safety of folate supplementation have been expressed. Pernicious anemia can be masked (allowing vitamin B12 deficiency to progress); zinc function can be disrupted; and concurrent medications, such as Dilantin, can be antagonized (Hathcock, 1997). Although some studies suggest that supplemental folic acid can affect zinc nutriture, others demonstrate no evidence of this (Kauwell, Bailey, Gregory, Bowling, & Cousins, 1995).

The current recommendation (RDA) of folate is 180 micromg per day, and for vitamin B6 it is 1.6 mg per day. Recommended foods include cereals fortified with folic acid (Malinow et al., 1998). In U.S. food supplies, folate is supplemented to grain products in the amount of 140 micromg per 100 g of grain; even after fortification, the majority of individuals will have folate intake below that which is beneficial (Tucker, Mahnken, Wilson, Jacques, & Selhub, 1996).

Vitamin A. Adequate plasma retinol, or vitamin A, levels appear to be maintained in older people. Although many elderly take supplements that contain vitamin A, data suggest that due to an increase in absorption from the gastrointestinal tract and a decrease in hepatic uptake, vitamin A is one of the only nutrients in which requirements decrease with advancing age (Lipschitz, 1995). Side effects of vitamin A toxicity include headaches, lassitude, reduction in white cell counts, impaired hepatic function, and bone pain.

Vitamin A and beta carotene have been suggested as exerting a protective effect against the development of neoplasms. Recent large-scale controlled trials have failed to prove definitively a beneficial effect of beta carotene in reducing the risk of the development of skin cancers.

Vitamin D. Recent studies suggest that vitamin D deficiency may be a serious concern in older people, with 62% to 72% below the RDA (McCormack, 1997). Whether age influences vitamin D absorption from the gastrointestinal tract is not clear. Seasonal variations in serum vitamin D levels are greater in lean than in fat participants. Sunshine appears to be an important factor in maintaining appropriate vitamin D status in older people. Lack of adequate vitamin D and calcium are associated with osteoporosis and osteomalacia. A negative correlation has been found between vitamin D intake and fractures. Vitamin D may help in healing skin lesions, especially psoriasis, and actinic keratoses (Holick, 1994). Vitamin D deficiency increases susceptibility to the development of pulmonary tuberculosis by compromising macrophage function. In any patient with severe osteoporosis, fracture, or bone pain, vitamin D-induced osteomalacia must be excluded.

Vitamin E. The tocopherols are lipophilic compounds, and they demonstrate their antioxidant properties in membrane tissue or in lipoprotein particles. They exert their action on lipid peroxyl radicals, generating intermediate biochemical compounds that are less toxic to PUFAs (Stahl & Sies, 1997). Dietary sources of vitamin E may be found in vegetable oils (soybean, corn, cottonseed, virgin olive oils, and safflower) and products made from these oils, such as margarine or mayonnaise. Wheat germ is one of the best sources, and nuts and some leafy green vegetables are desirable sources. The minimum amount of vitamin E needed to protect PUFAs against oxidative damage is at least 0.4 to 0.8 mg per gram of PUFAs, and may be in excess of 1.5 mg/g if the individual diet is characterized by an excess of PUFAs (Weber, Bendich, & Machlin, 1997).

Vitamin E supplements provide independent protective effects for all-cause mortality and for CHD mortality, lowering total mortality rates by 27%, reducing the risk of heart disease mortality by 41%, and decreasing cancer mortality by 22% (Jha, Flather, Lonn, Farkouh, & Yusuf, 1995). Data substantiate that those individuals having higher blood levels and dietary intakes of vitamin E have significantly lower CHD rates and decreased risk of heart attack in both men and women (Jha et al., 1995). In postmenopausal women, an inverse relation was found between the intake of vitamin E (from food sources) and risk of death from CHD; intake of vitamins A and C did not appear to be associated with reduced risk. Vitamin E intake also was associated with a more healthful cardiovascular risk profile (Kushi et al., 1996).

Two large prospective trials (39,910 male health professionals, 87,245 female nurses) found that individuals who used vitamin E supplements daily for at least 2 years had 40% lower rates of CHD and significantly less atherosclerosis compared to those who consumed less of the vitamin (Stampfer et al., 1993). Short-duration doses and doses less than 100 IU had no effect. Similarly, in patients with diagnosed CHD, doses of 400 to 800 IU of vitamin E daily for more than 1 year led to significantly lower risk of a subsequent nonfatal myocardial infarction (Weber et al., 1997).

Vitamin E intakes, much higher than the current recommendations, have been shown to significantly reduce oxidative alterations of LDLs. In one study, 1,000 IU of vitamin E given for 7 days resulted in a 41% increase in oxidative resistance of LDLs (Esterbauer, Dieber-Rotheneder, Striegel, & Waeg, 1991). Platelet adherence to an injured blood vessel wall is thought to be the first step in platelet-induced thrombus formation (Opie, 1997). Vitamin E affects platelet adhesion in a dose-dependent manner (Jandak, Steiner, & Richardson, 1989). In healthy volunteers, 2 weeks of 200 IU of vitamin E led to a decrease in platelet adherence of 44%; 2 additional weeks of supplementation resulted in additional decrease in platelet adherence of 77% (Steiner, 1993). Most literature suggests that the antioxidant vitamin E is strongly related to reduced risk of CHD; the vitamin also has a wide safety margin. There is evidence that supplements of 200 to 2,400 IU/day (13-160 times the RDA) for a period of 4.5 years were safe (Kappus & Diplock, 1992).

Vitamin E (alpha-tocopherol) is abundant in the diet, and deficiencies of the vitamin are rare. It is involved in the function of the enzyme glutathione peroxidase, which is involved in free radical generation. The vitamin also affects the biophysical properties of the cell membrane, reducing the age-related increase in membrane microviscosity. Vitamin E also influences immune function, and recent evidence indicates that administration of the vitamin enhances immune function in older people and may minimize infectious risk. Some of the most intriguing data involve the effects of vitamin E administration on immune function in old experimental animals and, more recently, in older men and women.

The most dramatic demonstration of antioxidant effects was in a report by Chandra, Chandra, Agrawal, Ghatak, and Pandy (1994), who conducted a placebo-controlled, double-blind trial of supplementation of healthy older men and women with a multiple vitamin containing the RDA for most vitamins, with the exception of vitamin E and beta carotene, which were about four times the upper quartile of usual intakes. Supplementation was associated with marked increases in various parameters of immunity. The supplemented group had only half the number of days with infection and 60% of days taking antibiotics during the 1-year trial.

Data also substantiate that those individuals having higher blood levels and dietary intakes of vitamin E have significantly lower CHD rates and decreased risk of heart attack in both men and women (Stampfer et al., 1993). Hodis, Mack, and La Bree (1995) found that participants who took 100 IU or more of vitamin E daily exhibited significantly less progression of atherosclerosis compared to those who consumed less of the vitamin. Similarly, Stephens, Parsons, and Schofield (1996) found that in patients with diagnosed CHD, doses of 400 to 800 IU of vitamin E daily for over 1 year led to significantly lower risk of a subsequent nonfatal myocardial infarction. Losonczy, Harris, and Havlik (1996) found independent protective effects of vitamin E supplements for all-cause mortality and for CHD mortality. Vitamin E supplements were found to lower total mortality rates by 27%, reduce the risk of heart disease mortality by 41%, and decrease cancer mortality by 22%.

Beta carotene. Carotenoids, which are precursors to vitamin A, are natural colorants with significant antioxidant activity. They scavenge peroxyl radicals by chemical interaction (Stahl & Sies, 1997). Some of the major food sources of carotenoids are carrots, tomatoes, citrus fruits, and spinach. High doses of beta carotene are well tolerated; very high (> 30 mg/day) doses are related to skin discoloration related to hypercarotenemia. Supplemental dosages of 25 mg each day have been recommended as safe for most adults (Hathcock, 1997).

Several studies have been conducted examining the efficacy of beta carotene in CHD risk reduction: the Physician's Health Study (Buring et al.,
1995); the Carotenoid and Retinol Efficacy Trial (Omenn et al., 1996); and
the Alpha-Tocopherol, Beta Carotene Cancer Prevention Study Group
(1994). These studies failed to find any benefit in beta carotene supplementation; indeed, significant increases of cancer in the "high-risk" population
were found; however, those trials were of short duration or had samples at
high risk for cancer.

In the Health Professionals Study (39,000 men), participants in the highest quintile of carotene from dietary intake (19,034 IU/day) had a 4.8-fold
reduction in relative risk for an AMI, compared to those in the lowest quintile
(Jha et al., 1995). This observation also was demonstrated in the Lipid
Research Clinic's follow-up study of men with type IIA hyperlipidemia.
Patients in the highest quartile of serum carotenoid levels had a 36% reduction in risk (Morris, Kritchevsky, & Davis, 1994). Other studies show an
association of an increased consumption of beta carotene with a decreased
risk of cancer (Van Poppel & Goldbohm, 1995). This effect is attributed to
the antioxidant properties of beta carotene that inhibit factors in the early
stages of cancer (Bertram & Bortkiewicz, 1995).

In the Iowa Women's Health Study (41,836 postmenopausal women),
it was found that vitamin E intake from food was inversely related to risk
of death from CHD (Kushi et al., 1996). These findings held even after
adjustment of age and dietary intake (Kushi et al., 1996).

Dreosti (1997) observed that studies demonstrating the value of the antioxidant vitamins in reducing the risk of certain degenerative diseases often
include supplementation of single vitamins at least ten times greater than is
feasible from dietary intake. Protective benefits have been observed when
dietary intakes of fruits and vegetables occur at only two to three times current RDAs, due to the complexity of the antioxidant defense system and the
interactive effect of these combinations. The safety and efficacy of higher-
dose antioxidants has yet to be demonstrated.

Fish oil. N-3 fatty acids are important components of all cell membranes,
and they have anti-inflammatory effects (Mori, Beilin, Burke, Morris, &
Ritchie, 1997). It is hypothesized that very long chain n-3 PUFAs of fish oil
have a positive effect on lipid metabolism and the hemostatic system. In a
randomized, placebo-controlled study ($N = 47$ men), fish oil was associated
with a 30% decline in plasma triglycerides (Marckmann, Bladbierg, &
Jespersen, 1997). The information available concerning the efficacy of fish
oil supplementation has been determined only among male patients.

Most prospective cohort studies report inverse associations between fish consumption and cardiovascular mortality (Daviglus et al., 1997; Kromhout, Feskens, & Bowles, 1995). It is hypothesized that this effect is accomplished through decreasing the incidence of fatal arrhythmia. Experimental data suggest that the n-3 fatty acids in fish have antiarrhythmic properties and are associated with a 50% reduction in primary cardiac arrest (Siscovick et al., 1995). In the Physician's Health Study (20,551 U.S. male physicians, followed for 11 years), participants who consumed one fish meal a week had a relative risk of sudden death of .48, compared to those who consumed fish less than monthly (Albert et al., 1998).

Vitamin K. Vitamin K is essential for the production of a number of factors involved in both the intrinsic and extrinsic clotting cascade. There is evidence that vitamin K administration is beneficial in elderly people who have an explained prolongation of their prothrombin time. Although dietary intake is adequate, deficiencies can result from the administration of drugs that interfere with the vitamin's absorption or interfere with bacterial flora. The recommended adequate intake of vitamins is found in Table 4.3.

Mineral Requirements

Numerous studies indicate that, for a wide variety of minerals and vitamins, intake is significantly lower than the RDA for a large proportion of ambulatory elderly (Chernoff, 1995). However, as lean body mass decreases with age, the requirement for trace elements needed for muscle metabolism may be reduced (Chernoff & Lipschitz, 1985).

Calcium. Calcium has a role in promoting increased peak bone mass and delaying the onset of osteoporosis (Hathcock, 1997). Sufficient calcium intake during early adulthood increases peak bone mass, reducing the risk of osteoporosis in later life (Hathcock, 1997). Calcium is absorbed by active transport and passive diffusion across the intestinal mucosa. Fractional calcium absorption varies inversely with daily calcium intake. In postmenopausal women, fractional calcium absorption declines about 21% per year (NIH Consensus Statement, 1993). In elderly women, bone loss due to osteoporosis, the presence of hypochlorhydria, and the attendant failure to absorb calcium efficiently suggests the need for additional calcium supplementation.

It is generally recommended that calcium intake in older people be between 1.0 and 1.3 g per day to slow the decline of bone density (NIH Consensus Statement, 1993). The efficiency of the absorption of calcium

(Text continued on page 98)

TABLE 4.3 Vitamins

Vitamin	Dose	Action	Evidence of Alteration	Reference
A	1,000 mg retinol equivalents for men; 800 mg retinol equivalents for women	Protective effect against the development of neoplasms	Excess: headaches, lassitude, reduction in white cell counts, impaired hepatic function, bone pain	Suter (1991)
Beta carotene (precursors to vitamin A)	25 mg/day	Scavenge peroxyl radicals, protective effect against the development of neoplasms		Hathcock (1997); Stahl & Sies (1997)
B[1] Thiamine[a]	1.1–1.2 mg/d (RDAs)	Carbohydrate metabolism	Deficiency is common in alcoholics, contributing factor in the development of disordered cognition, neuropathies, and cardiomyopathies	Food and Nutrition Board, 1998; Pitkin, 1998; Suter, 1991
B[2] Riboflavin[a]	1.2 mg/day (RDA) for men; 1.1 mg/day (RDA) for women	Electron transfer reactions	Deficiency: ariboflavinosis	Food and Nutrition Board (1998); Pitkin (1998); Suter (1991)
B[6]	1.7 mg/day (AI) for men; 1.5 mg/day (AI) for women	Metabolism of amino acids, degradation of tryptophan, breakdown of glycogen to glucose-1-phosphate	Deficiency seen in alcoholics	Food and Nutrition Board (1998); Pitkin (1998); Suter (1991)

B[12]	2.4 mcg/day (foods fortified with B[12] or B[12]-containing supplement) (RDAs)	Prevent decline in cognitive function associated with aging	Deficiency: pernicious anemia, severe megaloblastic anemia, gait disorders, sensory and motor neurologic deficits, and memory loss, poor immune response, loss of gastric intrinsic factor	Food and Nutrition Board (1998); Pitkin (1998); Rosenberg & Miller (1992)
Biotin	30 mcg/day (AI)	Cofactor in metabolism of fatty acids and the deamination of certain amino acids	Deficiency seen in long-term parenteral nutrition	Food and Nutrition Board (1998); Pitkin (1998)
C[a]	60 mg/day (megadoses have no clinical value); 100 mg/day in cigarette smokers	Prevents the oxidation of low-density lipoprotein, preserves vitamin E and beta carotene levels during oxidative stress, retards the development of atherosclerosis, alters the metabolism of cholesterol, affects triglyceride levels through modulation of lipoprotein lipase activity, decreases the propensity of platelets to adhere to the vessel wall; improves the rate of wound healing	Deficiency: lassitude, fatigue, purpura, capillary hemorrhaging, bleeding from the gums, delayed wound healing	Enstrom, Kanim, & Klein (1992); Gey (1998); Lynch et al. (1996); Stahl & Sies (1997); Suter (1991)

(Continued)

TABLE 4.3 Continued

Vitamin	Dose	Action	Evidence of Alteration	Reference
Choline	550 mg/day (AI) for men; 425 mg/day (AI) for women	Prevents the deposit of fat in the liver, is essential in synaptic transmission of nerve impulses		Food and Nutrition Board (1998); Pitkin (1998); Suter (1991)
D[a]	10-15 mg/day (in absence of sunlight exposure); as cholecalciferol, 1 mcg = 40 IU of vitamin D (AIs)	Heals skin lesions, especially psoriasis, and actinic keratoses	Deficit: osteoporosis, osteomalacia, fractures, increases susceptibility to TB	Food and Nutrition Board (1998); Holick (1994); Pitkin (1998); McCormack (1997)
E (tocopherols and lipophilic compounds)	0.4-0.8 mg/g of PUFAs, 400-800 IU, and 200-2,400 IU/day (13-160 times the RDA) for a period of 4.5 years were safe	Antioxidant properties, reducing coronary heart disease risk, decrease in platelet adherence, improves cell-mediated immunity, increases in various parameters of immunity	Deficiency is rare except in severe cases of malabsorption	Jha et al. (1995); Kappus & Diplock (1992); Kushi et al. (1996); Rimm et al. (1993); Stahl & Sies (1997); Stampfer et al. (1993); Steiner (1993); Suter (1991); Weber et al. (1997)

Nutrient	Recommended Intake	Function	Deficiency/Excess	References
Folate	400 cg/day (1 mcg food folate = 0.6 mcg of folic acid = 0.5 mcg synthetic folic acid) (RDAs)	Transport of single carbon atoms in intermediary metabolic processes	Deficiency in the elderly is predominantly found in alcoholics; may result in cognitive loss or significant depression. Excess: masks pernicious anemia; disrupts zinc function; antagonizes concurrent medications (Dilantin)	Food and Nutrition Board (1998); Hathcock (1997); Pitkin (1998); Suter (1991)
Niacin	16 mg/day (RDA) for men; 14 mg/day (RDA) for women (Niacin equivalents: 1 mg niacin = 60 mg tryptophan coenzyme component)	Constituent of the redox coenzymes NAD and NADP	Dermatitis, inflammation of mucous membranes, diarrhea, and psychic disturbances (pellagra)	Food and Nutrition Board (1998); Pitkin (1998); Suter (1991)
K	1 mcg/kg	Production of clotting factors	Bleeding	Suter (1991)
Panothenic acid	5 mg/day (AI)			Food and Nutrition Board (1998); Pitkin (1998); Suter (1991)

NOTE: RDA = recommended dietary allowance (dietary intake sufficient to meet the requirement of nearly all—97% to 98%—healthy people in a particular life stage and gender group). AI = adequate intake (AI is based on observed or experimentally determined estimates of nutrient intake by a group of healthy people).
a. Inadequate dietary intake in the elderly.

97

from supplements is greatest when calcium is taken in doses of 500 mg or less, taken with dietary fats (NIH Consensus Statement, 1993). In food sources of calcium, the calcium content varies; in comparison with calcium from milk, calcium from dried beans is about half, with spinach about one tenth.

Population studies also have indicated an inverse relation between calcium intake and the prevalence of hypertension (Morris & McCarron, 1987). Population studies indicate that the relation between dietary calcium intake and systolic blood pressure is independent of age, gender, race, socioeconomic status, geography, and body weight (McCarron, Morris, Young, Roullet, & Drueke, 1991). Although meta-analysis of randomized clinical trials concluded that the reduction in systolic blood pressure is not sufficient to warrant calcium supplementation for hypertension prevention or treatment (Allender et al., 1996), certain population groups, such as hypertensive, diabetic African Americans, may benefit from increased calcium intake (Zemel, Zemel, Bryg, & Sowers, 1990).

Zinc. The prevalence of zinc deficiency is important because of the role that this mineral plays in food intake and in wound healing. In elderly participants with chronic debilitating diseases, modest zinc deficiency may contribute to anorexia. There is also evidence that zinc supplementation aids in wound healing in general and in the healing of pressure ulcers in particular (Allman, 1989). Zinc supplementation also has been shown to improve immune function and impede the rate of development of macular degeneration in older people. Intakes of zinc in older people decline in relation to the decrease in energy intake and are much lower than the recommended level of 15 mg/day for men and 12 mg/day for women. Low plasma zinc concentrations have been found in 2% to 27% of the elderly population (Bogden et al., 1987). Zinc deficiency is associated with impaired immune function, anorexia, delayed wound healing, and pressure sore development.

Iron. Aging is associated with a gradual increase in iron stores in both men and women. As a consequence, iron deficiency is rare in older people and invariably is caused by pathologic blood loss. It is important to emphasize that the anemia of chronic disease, which is associated with iron-deficient erythropoiesis, including a low serum iron concentration and a reduced transferrin saturation, is frequently misdiagnosed as iron-deficient anemia in older people. This results in the inappropriate administration of oral iron therapy and unnecessary invasive investigative procedures to identify the source of iron loss.

Recent studies indicate a correlation between increased iron stores and risks of neoplasia and CAD. Because aging is associated with increasing iron stores, supplementation with oral iron may not be desirable in older persons. Anemia in older people is usually related to blood loss, often from the gastrointestinal tract, and requires medical attention.

Selenium. There is suggestive evidence that selenium deficiency may contribute to age-related declines in cellular function. The mineral may be involved in minimizing free radical accumulation, because it is essential for the normal function of glutathione peroxidase. Significant selenium deficiency is rare. There is some evidence that selenium deficiency may contribute to a greater neoplastic risk and declines in immune function. Furthermore, selenium deficiency has been associated with a two- to threefold risk of CHD mortality (Salonen, Alfthan, Huttunen, Pikkarainen, & Puska, 1982) and is correlated with coronary atherosclerosis (Moore, Noiva, & Wells, 1984).

Copper. Generally, aging is associated with increases in serum copper concentrations, although the significance of this increase is unknown. Copper deficiency is rare and has been reported in those patients receiving total parenteral nutrition.

Chromium. Recent evidence has suggested an important role for chromium in carbohydrate metabolism. Studies have shown age-related declines in tissue chromium levels. It is possible that chromium deficiency may contribute to glucose intolerance in older people, although the therapeutic efficacy of chromium replacement is controversial. The mineral and trace mineral requirements are presented in Tables 4.4 and 4.5.

Fluid Intake

Fluid balance is extremely important because of the propensity of older people to develop dehydration and the ease with which overhydration can occur in elderly individuals with compromised renal function or other disorders associated with fluid retention. Dehydration is the most common cause of fluid and electrolyte disturbances in older people (Chernoff, 1994); it significantly increases health care costs, and it is predictive of death within a year of admission for approximately half of older Medicare patients hospitalized (Chernoff, 1995).

Dehydration risk increases due to reduced thirst sensation and reduced fluid intake, along with diminished water conservation by the kidneys, de-

TABLE 4.4 Mineral Requirements

Mineral	Dose	Action	Reference
Calcium	1.2 g/day (AI)	Promoting increased peak bone mass, delaying the onset of osteoporosis	Food and Nutrition Board (1998); Hathcock (1997); Hoover et al. (1996); Pitkin (1998)
Phospherous	700 mg/day (RDA)	Helps in bone formation and maintenance, important in metabolism of ATP	Food and Nutrition Board (1998); Fosmire (1991); Lindeman & Beck (1991); Pitkin (1998)
Magnesium	420 mg/day (RDA) for men; 320 mg/day (RDA) for women	Important intracellular cation acts as activator for many enzymes	Food and Nutrition Board (1998); Fosmire (1991); Lindeman & Beck (1991); Pitkin (1998)

NOTE: AI = adequate intake (AI is based on observed or experimentally determined estimates of nutrient intake by a group of healthy people). RDA = recommended dietary allowance (dietary intake sufficient to meet the requirement of nearly all—97% to 98%—healthy people in a particular life stage and gender group).

creased renin activity and aldosterone secretion, and medication side effects (Weinberg & Minaker, 1995). As a general rule, water intake should be 1 ml/kcal or 30 ml/kg body weight. Dehydration may be the most common cause of an acute confusional state in older people (Lipschitz, 1995). This is primarily related to the age-related decline in thirst drive. Studies have demonstrated a decreased ability of older people to respond to fluid deprivation. This becomes a particularly serious problem in frail elderly who develop minor infections or illness. This results in fever, increased metabolism, and fluid loss. Thus, aggressive attempts at assuring adequate hydration are essential in older people. Patients and their families must be educated to emphasize the importance of maintaining adequate fluid intake at all times and to monitor intake if a minor illness develops or if fluid requirements are increased, such as during outdoor activities in the summer.

TABLE 4.5 Mineral Requirements: Trace Metals

Mineral (Trace Metal)	Dose	Action	Reference
Chromium	Controversial; 50-100 mcg/day	Role in carbohydrate metabolism, deficiency may contribute to glucose intolerance	Fosmire (1991)
Copper	RDA not established; 1.5-3.0 mg/day	Essential in proper bone metabolism, prevention of skeletal abnormality; deficiency is rare and has been reported in patients receiving total parenteral nutrition	Fosmire (1991)
Selenium	70 mcg/day (RDA) for men; 55 mcg/day (RDA) for women	Minimizing free radical accumulation, essential for the normal function of glutathione peroxidase, optimal immune function, decreased risk of coronary atherosclerosis	Fosmire (1991); Moore et al. (1984); Salonent et al. (1982)
Zinc	15 mg/day for men; 12 mg/day for women	Factor in DNA synthesis; aids in wound healing, improves immune function, impedes macular degeneration	Allman (1989); Bogden et al. (1987); Fosmire (1991)

NOTE: AI = adequate intake (AI is based on observed or experimentally determined estimates of nutrient intake by a group of healthy people). RDA = recommended dietary allowance (dietary intake sufficient to meet the requirement of nearly all—97% to 98%—healthy people in a particular life stage and gender group).

Managing Nutritional Status

Factors affecting nutritional status are multidimensional and interrelated at any age. Measures to promote good nutrition must specifically address the needs and problems of older adults to be effective.

Overnutrition. Preliminary data from animal studies has indicated that life expectancy can be significantly extended by restricting food intake. Masoro

(1993) indicated that caloric restriction leads to longer life in rodents. Furthermore, animal studies have shown that nutritional deprivation delays maturation and significantly prolongs life expectancy (McCarter, 1995). These investigations have shown that caloric restriction causes delays in bio-markers of aging and results in leaner and more active animals. Weindruch and Sohal (1997) found that initiating caloric restriction in rats reduced the rate of muscle degeneration of protected muscle mitochondrial genome. However, the mechanism by which food restriction results in prolongation of life span is still not clear. A study examining the human response to calo-ric restriction found that over a period of 15 years, all-cause mortality was highest in men who were very thin (BMI less than 20) or very fat (BMI higher than 30). The risk of cardiovascular disease, myocardial infarction, and dia-betes mellitus was lowest in men with BMIs between 20 and 24 (Jebb, 1997).

For individuals between age 60 and 70 who are healthy and ambulatory but significantly overweight, hypercholesterolemic, or hypertensive, an effort to reduce calories, fat, and sodium intake is warranted. Given the difficulties of weight loss, high rates of weight regain, and potential dangers of weight cycling, primary prevention of obesity remains the optimal approach to mini-mizing obesity-related health risks.

Several ethnic-minority groups are at particularly high risk for obesity (Kumanyika, 1990). Cultural differences, educational attainment (Kahn, Williamson, & Stevens, 1991), economic factors, and differences in physical activity and in perceptions about health risk all may contribute to risk of weight gain (Wing, Matthews, Kuller, Meilahn, & Plantinga, 1991). Pre-vention efforts should be targeted particularly at these higher-risk groups. Efforts aimed at individuals, families, and communities may be appropriate. The primary health care provider plays an important role not only in treating obesity and its complications but also in identifying and educating those at risk.

For patients who are overweight, a diet with fewer total calories from fat and an increase in physical activity should be recommended. In general, the goal should be a weight loss of from one half pound to 1 pound per week. Although more rapid weight loss may be achieved with a very low-calorie (800 kcal/day or less) diet, weight loss from these diets usually is not well maintained and may lead to health problems. The food guide pyramid may be used as a basis for dietary instruction and menu planning to promote weight loss. Selected patients who have failed at conservative methods of weight loss and who are severely obese or have obesity-related medical problems may benefit from the short-term weight loss of very low calorie diets, under medical supervision. A diet of less than 30% fat, high in complex carbohydrates, and low in simple sugars can be recommended generally for older persons. However, dietary approaches alone do not reduce weight in overweight persons (Wood, Stefanick, Williams, & Haskell, 1991).

Behavior therapy and increased physical activity have been shown to help initiate and maintain efforts at weight loss. Combined with dietary modification, a program of moderate, regular physical activity promotes weight loss and maintains lean body mass. Behavior modification techniques for weight reduction include self-monitoring activities, stimulus control, and self-rewards for goal achievement. Self-monitoring may include keeping a food diary of what foods are eaten, how much is eaten, where food is eaten, and the emotional circumstances surrounding consumption. This information may be used to identify specific environmental or emotional cues for eating behaviors, including overeating, and outline strategies for effective behavioral change. Stimulus control techniques include control of self and the environment to facilitate weight loss. Examples include removing high-fat foods from the home, not eating while watching television, and eating at designated times. Self-reward provides positive reinforcement for goal achievement. Rewards are determined by the individual for specific behavioral and weight loss goals and should not include food items.

MANAGEMENT OF STRESSORS

Health Promotion Interventions in Ethnically Diverse Elderly

The recognition that gender, racial, and ethnic factors play an important role in the health risks and health promotion behaviors of vulnerable elderly individuals, particularly women, is an important one. Ethnicity influences health, health beliefs and behavior, and relationships with health care professionals (Hopper, 1993). Health practitioners who work with vulnerable populations may benefit from a deep understanding of particular cultural values and beliefs that influence health behavior.

The new awareness of diversity in the United States has a profound effect on all aspects of society; cultural limitations of intervention models are no longer functional in this changing environment. Ethnic and gender identity is part of a cultural system of shared beliefs, customs, and values, and these elements should be used to identify strategies specific to the health promotion of vulnerable groups.

Health promotion efforts among cultural groups require that health care providers develop intervention strategies that are culturally meaningful and appropriate to the target group. Culturally competent models incorporate the values and ideologies underpinning the target culture. All too often, intervention strategies for health promotion are based on models that have been successful in mainstream (white) communities. The use of culturally inappropriate models has led to the creation of cultural gaps between recommended behavior and the individual's ability or willingness to adopt the behavior (Coalition of Hispanic Health and Human Services Organizations [COSSMHO], 1995). Access to prevention and treatment may be reduced as a result of poor fit between the delivery of care and culturally acceptable systems. Characteristics essential to the provision of culturally relevant health promotion efforts to vulnerable groups include communication, family and kinship networks, and access to and acceptance of medical involvement in health matters.

Communication. A critical factor in health promotion efforts is establishing or improving communication with the cultural groups. Communication is the core of a health promotion intervention, and knowledge of cultural differences in communication is paramount to program success. Communication style among diverse groups is perhaps the most salient of cultural differences (Hecht, Collier, & Ribeau, 1993). Many authors report that the identification of appropriate spokespersons can contribute to program success (Sallis et al., 1988). Williams and Flora (1995) found that health promotion behavior changes related to cardiovascular risk (smoking, diet, and exercise) varied according to segments of the population. For example, among Spanish-speaking individuals, the less acculturated, less educated, older groups were more accessible by Spanish-language television communication, whereas the more acculturated, more educated groups could be reached through the English language media, including newspapers. Targeted communication of health messages helped disseminate culturally relevant health messages to reach population segments with specific attitudes, behaviors, and preferences.

Understanding cultural explanations of health and illness can assist the provider in developing relevant strategies for risk modification. Knowledge and use of cultural expressions, idioms, and differences associated with language and modes of expression used in a culture will enhance the ability of the provider to communicate effectively and influence behavior.

Family and kinship. In many non-Western cultures, the concept of the family extends beyond the "nuclear" family; there is frequently no distinction between the immediate and "extended" family. In these cultural groups, it is common for members of the extended family to share a home and personal resources (COSSMHO, 1995). In the Hispanic culture, family members are relied on for emotional and spiritual help, more so than are external sources of support (COSSMHO, 1995). Although white Americans have been raised on the ethic of survival through self-reliance, African Americans have been raised on the ethic of survival through mutual aid and interdependence (Kumanyika et al., 1992). In the white-American culture, the surrounding community is a loose social network rather than a primary source of reciprocal support, advice, and assistance (COSSMHO, 1995). In contrast, members of the Hispanic community interact with and rely on members of the surrounding community the same way Anglo-Americans rely on their extended family (COSSMHO, 1995). Among African American groups, the extended family and social networks in the culture have significant importance (Bailey, 1987; Kumanyika et al., 1992).

Deep spiritual feelings by individuals in certain cultural groups evidence a "sharing" of illness and "partnership" with God in the efforts to manage health promotion and prevention efforts. Church-based programs are particularly effective in the African American community because of the central role of churches in social, social support, and communication networks of this cultural group (Kerner, Dusenbury, & Mandelblatt, 1993).

Access to and acceptance of health interventions. Access to needed medical care and acceptance of therapeutic interventions may be dependent on a number of factors, including the presence of poverty. Acceptance of therapeutic interventions may depend on cultural issues, including perceptions of personal space, cultural values, and time orientation. Aspects of personal space, proximity, and distance hold different meanings among cultural groups. Physical closeness, exposure to private body parts, and discussion of intimate issues have unique variability in their acceptance across cultures.

Acknowledging and respecting private issues and personal values will enhance efforts to design culturally relevant interventions. For example, among African Americans, the value of adequate rest has been shown to be as important as, if not more important than, exercise or increased physical activity (Airhihenbuwa, Kumanyika, Agurs, & Lowe, 1995). The health care provider needs to explore cultural values concerning health promotion and prevention behaviors among vulnerable groups and develop strategies that would facilitate behavior that would be acceptable and successful.

Strategies to enhance access to and acceptance of culturally relevant intervention efforts include conducting focus groups in churches and community centers to establish a "place" for health promotion in the community. Church and community sites can be used as focal areas for teaching and screening efforts, recruiting participants through church-based activities, such as choir or bingo events.

Communication styles, manipulation of language, understanding language usage and idioms, and focusing on cultural groups can enhance communication of health promotion efforts. Family and kinship networks can provide important links in both the development and implementation of culturally relevant health promotion programs. Using family members to support and encourage health-promoting behavior can facilitate attendance at programs and health events and support risk modification efforts. Failure to understand and acknowledge cultural values often hampers efforts to facilitate health behavior changes among individuals and groups. An understanding of the burden that poverty creates can assist the health care provider to increase opportunities for the poor and disadvantaged to have access to health promotion efforts. Awareness of cultural variation has a profound effect on all aspects of health care, particularly health promotion. Health promotion and prevention efforts must be sensitive to and reflect the cultural and socioeconomic context of each individual.

MANAGEMENT OF CARDIOVASCULAR RISK

Hypertension

Among Americans aged 60 and over, hypertension is found in 60% of non-Hispanic whites, 71% of African Americans, and 61% of Mexican Americans (Joint National Committee VI, 1997). The most common form of hypertension among older people is primary hypertension, and treatment of hypertension in older people has shown major benefits. Treatment of isolated systolic hypertension in older people has been shown to decrease nonfatal infarction, left ventricular failure, and stroke over 4.5 years (SHEP Cooperative Research Group, 1991). Thus, attention to systolic blood pressure may be particularly important in older people.

The treatment of hypertension in older people should begin with lifestyle modification, such as weight loss and reduction of salt intake (Joint National Committee VI, 1997). If blood pressure changes are not achieved with lifestyle changes, pharmacologic therapy must be instituted. In the older individual, thiazide diuretics alone or in combination with beta-blockers are recommended (Frishman et al., 1994; SHEP Cooperative Research Group, 1991).

Appropriate assessment of the older individual with hypertension includes a thorough medical history, including duration of elevated blood pressure; family history of elevated blood pressure and heart disease; smoking or tobacco use; and dietary assessment, including intake of sodium and saturated fats. A history must be recorded of all medication use and of psychosocial and environmental factors that may influence blood pressure control (Joint National Committee VI, 1997). The physical examination should include serial blood pressure measurements separated by 2 minutes, with the individual supine or seated and after standing for at least 2 minutes; verification in the contralateral arm. In addition, a funduscopic examination, examination of the heart for rhythm abnormalities, murmurs, extrasystoles, the extremities for diminished or absent pulses, and the lungs for bronchospasm or adventitious sounds should be obtained.

Management of Unfavorable Lipids

Optimal serum cholesterol values for American adults should not exceed 200 mg/dl. Patients with an optimal blood cholesterol level should be provided with educational materials designed to maintain blood cholesterol levels below 200 mg/dl and reduce associated risk factors. These patients are advised to have another serum cholesterol test within 5 years. Serum cholesterol levels measuring 200 to 239 mg/dl are classified as "borderline high cholesterol." These patients are given dietary and associated risk factor modification guidelines designed to lower their serum cholesterol level and are rechecked annually. Individuals who have diagnosed CHD or two associated nonlipid risk factors need to be tested for serum, LDL-C, and HDL-C levels.

In addition to total blood cholesterol levels, the level of LDL cholesterol serves as a key index for clinical decision making in instituting cholesterol-lowering therapy. Desirable LDL cholesterol levels are 130 mg/dl and below. Levels of LDL cholesterol of 160 mg/dl or greater are classified as "high-risk," and those of 130 to 159 mg/dl are classified as "borderline high-risk." Patients with borderline high-risk LDL cholesterol are advised to follow a fat-modified diet and are reevaluated annually. Patients with diagnosed CHD or two associated nonlipid risk factors and all patients in the high-risk cholesterol group are evaluated annually and advised to enter cholesterol-lowering treatment programs. For secondary prevention in elderly adults with documented CHD, the optimal LDL cholesterol level is 100 mg/dl or less. When the LDL cholesterol level is above optimal, clinical evaluation is carried out and cholesterol-lowering therapy initiated. An HDL-C level of less than 35 mg/dl is defined as "low" and is considered a risk factor for CHD. Those people with HDL-C levels less than 35 mg/dl are advised to proceed to lipoprotein analysis.

Cholesterol reduction can be achieved by lifestyle changes including dietary therapy, weight loss, and physical activity, as well as a combination of lifestyle change and pharmacological therapy. People without high LDL cholesterol levels or severe dyslipidemias should be continued on dietary therapy for at least 6 months before considering drug therapy (NCEP, 1996). Modification of associated risk factors such as obesity, sedentary lifestyle, and smoking should be maintained throughout cholesterol-lowering therapy. If the goals of LDL cholesterol reduction are met by dietary modification, long-term monitoring is indicated. If reduction of LDL cholesterol is not achieved, lipid-lowering drugs are considered along with continued diet and exercise therapy.

Treatment goals for pharmacological therapy are the same as those used for dietary therapy. Both treatment modalities attempt to achieve LDL cholesterol levels of less than 160 mg/dl in patients without diagnosed CHD or two associated CHD risk factors, or LDL cholesterol levels of less than 130 mg/dl in patients with diagnosed CHD or two associated CHD risk factors. Guidelines established by the National Cholesterol Education Program (1996) recommend bile acid sequestrants and nicotinic acid as first-choice drugs for treatment of elevated levels of LDL. Both drugs are effective in lowering LDL cholesterol and have been found to lower CAD risk. Nicotinic acid is the drug of choice for patients with triglyceride levels of greater than 250 mg/dl because it lowers LDL cholesterol without exacerbating the hypertriglyceridemia. Administration of bile acid sequestrants may increase hepatic VLDL-C production and increase the plasma concentration of triglycerides. Bile acid sequestrants are thus contraindicated as single-drug therapy in patients with hypertriglyceridemia. Lovastatin is effective in lowering LDL cholesterol levels and produces a slight reduction in serum triglyceride levels. Fibric acid derivatives enhance lipoprotein lipase activity and hepatic bile secretion and reduce hepatic triglyceride production. Fibric acids appear to lower serum levels of VLDL-C and LDL-C and raise HDL-C levels. Thus, the net effect is to reduce the total cholesterol-HDL ratio.

The management of hyperlipidemia must incorporate a multifaceted approach composed of dietary modification, weight loss, exercise, and pharmacological therapy. For maximum reduction of CHD morbidity and mortality, all modifiable risk factors must be addressed. The overall objective in cholesterol reduction is to implement an individualized program leading to permanent lifestyle change. Both dietary and pharmacological therapy requires long-term behavioral changes. Adherence to lifestyle changes may be increased through a combination of education and behavior modification strategies.

When lipid values do not fall within appropriate guidelines, then nutrition, weight loss, and physical activity recommendations should be reevaluated. Based on the presence or absence of other risk factors, more extensive testing and follow-up are also recommended. If initial lipid values are elevated, plans are made to repeat the test within a few months. Following appropriate dietary and physical activity changes, individuals who show repeated elevations in total cholesterol and low levels of HDL-C should be considered for further evaluation, follow-up, and pharmacological therapy.

Control of Hyperglycemia

Because the control of hyperglycemia alone does not appear to reduce the risk of microvascular sequelae in people with diabetes mellitus, attention must be directed toward the management of associated cardiovascular risk factors. Risk reduction in the diabetic patient must begin with an assessment of patient needs and education related to the diabetic process and the role of associated risk factors (Fain, 1999). The primary factor in reduction of cardiovascular risk is dietary control. In the diabetic elderly, caloric restriction combined with intake alteration can significantly decrease plasma insulin, triglycerides, total cholesterol, VLDL-C, and elevated blood pressure; it also can increase HDL-C levels and aid in glycemic control. American Diabetes Association (1989) guidelines for dietary modification urge reduction in saturated fat and cholesterol intake and increased intake of dietary fiber and complex carbohydrates. These recommendations parallel those of the American Heart Association for prevention of CHD in the general population. Education and intervention for the diabetic patient must include a reduction of caloric intake to reduce the risk of CHD due to obesity. The increased risk of CHD in the obese elderly is the result of its association with atherogenic factors, such as hypertension, hypercholesterolemia, hypertriglyceridemia, and hyperinsulinemia.

Polypharmacy

At present, little is known about how older people understand information about their medical conditions or the treatment alternatives available to them. Reducing the burden of drugs taken by older persons wherever possible is important, because prescribing practices in the community and nursing homes may put older persons at risk (Gurwitz & Avorn, 1991; Willcox, Himmlestein, & Woolhandler, 1994). In older adults, consideration should be given to prescribing the fewest number of necessary drugs at the lowest initial dosage of medication possible, to reduce the risk of adverse effects. Providers may reduce adverse effects by prescribing the fewest number of drugs possible and simplifying the medication regimen. Brummel-Smith (1998) recommended treating each medical problem specifically for a given diagnosis. Each patient contact should be viewed as an opportunity to evaluate and, if appropriate, reduce the number of drugs taken. Colley and Lucas (1993) outlined a number of steps designed to simplify the medication regimen, including the elimination of pharmacological duplication, decrease of dosing frequency, and regular review of all drug regimens.

Patient education on prescription and over-the-counter drug reactions and interactions is essential. Medication side effects and symptoms of toxicity should be clearly outlined for patients and caretakers. Evaluation of potential medication interactions is essential, particularly during changes in prescription and dosage (Monane, Monane, & Selma, 1997). Frequent evaluations of medication use are recommended, as is the creation and use of an up-to-date list of medications with dosage and use schedules. A "brown bag" evaluation—in which all medications are bought to a care provider to identify what medications are taken for which symptoms and on what schedule—can reduce the risk of adverse reactions (Nolan & O'Malley, 1988). Medication evaluation should include prescription medications as well as over-the-counter drugs. Although research has shown that older people do have high rates of nonadherence related to drug use, with the help of external supports, adherence can be raised to the level exhibited by younger adults. Support measures may include systems of reminders to take medication as well as assistance by care providers or family members in organizing medication dosage and schedules through weekly medication dispensers.

Management of Hormone Alterations

Hormone replacement is one therapy that has application both in the alleviation of symptoms and as a preventive measure for a substantial number of conditions that affect elderly women of all cultures and all socioeconomic strata. However, many women have declined to initiate or to remain compliant with hormone replacement therapy (HRT).

The serious concern with estrogen replacement therapy is the potential increased risk of breast cancer. Although the protective effects of estrogen in CHD are unequivocal, CHD occurs later in life, whereas breast cancer occurs earlier, before age 65 (Lindsay et al., 1996). The correlation between the use of endogenous estrogen and the incidence of breast cancer is difficult to assess, due to differences in exposure time to estrogen and difficulty in relating biomarkers (estradiol) to biological effects in breast and bone tissue (Cauley et al., 1996). In some studies, the use of postmenopausal estrogen has been associated with an increased risk of breast cancer (Colditz et al., 1995).

However, these findings are inconsistent (Garland, Friedlander, Barrett-Connor, & Khaw, 1992; Kaufman et al., 1991; Speroff, 1996). Along with the length of exposure to exogenous estrogen, few studies differentiate between the past use and current use of the hormone and their relation to breast cancer incidence (Colditz, Egan, & Stampfer, 1993). The major concern in the interpretation of the studies is methodological: Short-term studies have been used to estimate long-term risks, and examinations of combined estrogen and progesterone therapy are relatively few (Colditz et al., 1993).

Several meta-analyses have addressed this problem and have yielded equivocal results, ranging from virtually no risk of breast cancer from the use of estrogen to a 30% increase in risk (Steinberg et al., 1991). The most recent analysis indicates that the relative risk of having breast cancer increased by a factor of 1.023 for each year of use among current users of HRT or those who ceased use 1 to 4 years previously (Collaborative Group on Hormonal Factors in Breast Cancer, 1997). The relative risk was 1.35 for women who had used HRT for 5 years or longer (average 11 years).

The risk of breast cancer does not appear to be increased with the combined use of estrogen and progestin (Stanford et al., 1995). A recent examination of long-term use of combination and estrogen-only therapy users documented no increase in the risk of breast cancer with either treatment (Newcomb et al., 1995).

In women with an intact uterus, the use of estrogen replacement therapy is strongly associated with significant risk of endometrial cancer, and there is almost certainly a causal relation (PEPI Writing Group, 1995; Weiss, 1996). The risk is further increased with prolonged use (an almost tenfold increased risk after 10 or more years of intake) and higher doses of estrogen. This increased risk is reversed following discontinuation of estrogens (Persson et al., 1992).

Reduction in the risk of endometrial hyperplasia is obtained by adding progesterone to estrogen replacement therapy. Studies have suggested that the addition of cyclic regimens of medroxyprogesterone are protective against endometrial hyperplasia (PEPI Writing Group, 1995). No increased risk is associated with women who add progesterone to the estrogen regimen. The risks of both ovarian and cervical cancer do not seem to be increased by use of HRT. However, available data are inconsistent (Persson et al., 1992).

Hormone Replacement Therapy as Prevention

The strongest argument for the use of estrogen replacement therapy is that the hormone exerts such favorable effects on CHD among postmenopausal women (Barrett-Connor & Bush, 1991; Lindsay et al., 1996; Stampfer & Colditz, 1991). The reduction in the development of CHD in women who used estrogen replacement is large: Some authors suggest 30% to 70%, others suggest 50% (Barrett-Connor & Bush, 1991; Stampfer & Colditz, 1991). Mortality from CHD is reported to be lower than among nonusers; however, the survival benefit diminishes with longer duration of use and is lower for women at low risk for coronary disease (Grodstein et al., 1997).

In the Cardiovascular Health Study (N = 2,955 women), both past and present estrogen use was associated with lower LDL-C, fibrinogen, glucose, insulin, and obesity, and with higher HDL-C and low levels of subclinical disease (Manolio et al., 1993). It has been shown that women with significant CHD who used estrogen had the same mortality as women with no coronary disease (Sullivan et al., 1990).

There are three mechanisms suggested to have primary responsibility for the favorable effects of estrogen on CHD. The first is a reduction in fibrinogen levels. Fibrinogen, a coagulation protein, has been shown to be an independent predictor of cardiovascular disease (Kannel, Wolf, Castelli, & D'Agostino, 1987). Although it is not clear whether fibrinogen is a casual risk factor or a marker for cerebrovascular disease (CVD), higher levels are found in both black and white women with known CVD and CHD (Folsom, Wu, Shahar, & Davis, 1993). Postmenopausal women using HRT have lower levels of fibrinogen than do nonusers. In the Postmenopausal Estrogen/ Progestin Intervention (PEPI) trial, higher fibrinogen levels were related to several physical and lifestyle characteristics—such as obesity, smoking, and both HDL-C and LDL-C—that are associated with the risk of CHD (Stefanick et al., 1995). It remains unclear whether fibrinogen is an independent risk factor for CHD.

Estrogen has well-documented overall effects on lipoproteins (the second protective mechanism; Udoff, Langenberg, & Adashi, 1995). After menopause, the LDL in women rises, surpassing that of men, reflecting estrogen deficiency (Barrett-Connor & Miller, 1993). LDL, the major atherogenic protein, carries about two thirds of the cholesterol and, combined with HDL, carries about 90% of plasma cholesterol.

Estrogen lowers LDL levels and increases HDL levels. The HDL attracts free cholesterol from the tissues and transports it to the liver for excretion, thus lowering plasma cholesterol (Nachtigall, Nachtigall, Nachtigall, & Beckman, 1979). Evidence from a large number of clinical trials documents significant decline in circulatory levels of LDL and rise in circulatory levels of HDL following HRT (Udoff et al.,1995). Combining the estrogen regimen with progestin to protect the endometrium against hyperplasia and cancer induced by estrogen appears to negate the rise in HDL. This negation of estrogen's ability to elevate HDL occurs with both cyclical and continuous regimens of progestin (Sherwin & Gelf, 1989). However, the 10-year study by Nachtigall et al. (1979) documented the sustained reduction of HDL/LDL ratios over that extended period. The dose of estrogen in that study was four times the current recommended dose. More recently, the PEPI trial results documented significant effects on lipids from combined regimens (PEPI Writing Group, 1995).

The third cardioprotective mechanism estrogen therapy offers is due to the action of the hormone on the endothelium and stabilization of the vascular system (Lindsay et al., 1996). In animal models, there is indication that estrogen has a direct effect on the reduction of coronary artery atheromas (Wagner et al., 1991). In women with angiographically documented CHD, those receiving estrogen replacement had significantly less coronary stenosis than those not receiving replacement (Sullivan et al., 1990). There is evidence that estrogen prevents vasoconstriction and may even increase blood flow (Wagner et al., 1991).

Data concerning the long-term beneficial effects of combination therapy are unavailable. The Heart and Estrogen-Progestin Replacement Study and the Women's Health Initiative assessing the effect of estrogen therapy on women with and without heart disease are under way (Lindsay et al., 1996).

Benefit of HRT on cognitive and affective functions. Estrogen may be an effective therapy for senile dementia in some older women (Schwartz, Freeman, & Frishman, 1995). Clinical studies examining women who have experienced surgical menopause demonstrate that menopause is associated with subclinical cognitive and affective dysfunction, both of which are improved by HRT. Long-term estrogen replacement may prevent late-life cognitive dysfunction. Clinical trials conducted among women with senile dementia have demonstrated substantial neurochemical effects, direct effects on vasculature, and effects on the generation of free radicals (Fillit, 1995). In the Atherosclerosis Risk in Communities study, a multicenter longitudinal investigation, estrogen replacement was associated with a higher performance on the "Word Fluency Test" of cognitive function. However, study participants ranged in age from 48 to 67, and this relatively younger mean age made these findings less generalizable to older elders, who experience a greater incidence of cognitive decline (Szklo et al., 1966).

In women diagnosed with impaired cognitive performance, such as that accompanying Alzheimer's disease, the results of estrogen replacement are more dramatic. Results of a matched comparison study indicated that women receiving estrogen performed significantly better on most neuropsychological tasks, particularly those tests examining memory, conceptualization, and visuopractical skills (Schmidt et al., 1996). Other studies that tested different cognitive-affective scales, such as the Mini-Mental State Examination, report similar findings (Ohkura et al., 1995).

Effects of HRT on osteoporosis. It has been estimated that estrogen replacement therapy and HRT may halve the risk of osteoporotic fractures in current users, although the risk of fracture is unaffected by relatively short-term use (Samsioe, 1997; Weiss, 1996). The effect on bone mass wears off after discontinuation of treatment but is never totally lost. It has been suggested that HRT could be started 15 to 20 years after the menopause and still provide protection for subsequent fractures (Lindsay et al., 1996). It is also known that estrogen affects calcium homeostasis, improves calcium absorption, and reduces calcium loss (Lindsay et al., 1996).

The controversy about hormone replacement exists because there is a substantial body of research that documents an association between HRT and the increased incidence of both breast and uterine cancer in women with an intact uterus. However, the favorable effects of estrogen on the prevention of osteoporosis, cognitive function, and CHD generate a complex therapeutic problem. The benefits of hormone therapy have been attributed in some instances to having used these therapies in the past, and in other instances, to long-term adherence (current use). Benefits have been observed to decrease over time because of the increase in mortality from breast cancer associated with long-term therapy (Grodstein et al., 1997).

Alternative Therapy for Hormone Alterations

Bioflavanoids. Phytoestrogens are naturally occurring sterols found in plants or their seeds. Isoflavones are plant sterol molecules (e.g., soy, garbanzo beans, legumes). Lignans are a constituent of the cell wall of plants and are made bioavailable through intestinal activity, after consumption of grains and seed oils (Murkies, Wilcox, & Davis, 1998; Taylor, 1997).

Recent research is focused on isoflavonoid phytoestrogens, the estrogenic plant chemicals found in soybeans and other legumes, which act as potent estrogen among postmenopausal women. These dietary sources of estrogen have been associated with decreased risks of breast cancer, reduced serum cholesterol, increased HDL, and beneficial effects on bone mineral density. Several bioflavanoid compounds have been identified; however, the main isoflavonoid phytoestrogens are equol (4,7-dihydroxyisoflavan and its precursor diadzein) and a metabolite of Biochanin A (5,7, dihydroxy-4, methoxyisoflavone) called genistein (4,5,7, trihydroxyisoflavone) (Adlercreutz et al., 1993; Verdeal & Ryan, 1979).

The isoflavones genistein and diadzein are reported to be weak estrogens, and they have been found to have the same pharmacologic efficacy equivalent to the biological hormone (Miksicek, 1993). In vitro studies in animal models (rats) have shown that naturally occurring phytoestrogens have estrogenic effects similar to endogenous estrogens and that they are conjugated within the system when given in human dietary concentrations (Adlercreutz et al., 1987).

Estrogenic flavonoids such as genistein demonstrate their mechanism of action through binding to estrogen receptor sites. They also have been noted for their ability to function as either estrogens or antiestrogens, depending on the biological environment and their chemical structures (Miksicek, 1993).

Phytoestrogens (genistein in particular) may act to inhibit cell growth and, therefore, the proliferation of hormone-dependent cancers, by binding to the estrogen-binding sites. Japanese women and women of Japanese origin in Hawaii who consume diets similar to the traditional Japanese diet, which is rich in soy products, have low breast cancer incidence and mortality (Adlercreutz et al., 1991).

Other studies have investigated the effect of phytoestrogens on the metabolism of sex hormone-binding globulin (SHBG) as a mechanism for the prevention of hormone-dependent cancers (Adlercreutz et al., 1987). Phytoestrogen consumption is associated with increased SHBG production in the liver. Production of higher SHBG levels decreases the concentration of bioavailable sex hormones, thus reducing their biological activity (Adlercreutz et al., 1987, 1991).

Limited evidence exists that use of phytoestrogens can have a beneficial effect on menopausal symptoms. In one small study of 58 postmenopausal women, those whose diets were supplemented with soy flour had a significant decrease in the number of hot flashes experienced per week, and menopausal symptoms also decreased significantly (Murkies et al., 1998). Another randomized clinical trial of 145 Israelis demonstrated an increase in SHBG among the 78 women who substituted phytoestrogen food sources for at least one fourth of their diet, and this increase in SHBG was associated with alleviation of hot flashes and urogenital symptoms (Brzezinski et al., 1997).

Phytoestrogens are thought to improve CHD risk by direct beneficial effect on the arterial vasculature and by inhibiting platelet aggregation, reducing serum cholesterol, or both. One 5-year prospective study of 805 older men (aged 65-84) demonstrated an inverse association between high intake of flavonoids consumed in a daily diet, including specific vegetables, fruits, and beverages (25.9 mg mean daily intake), and the incidence of myocardial infarction or mortality from CHD (Hertog, Fesdens, Hollman, Katan, & Kromhout, 1993).

Among peri- and postmenopausal women who participated in a double-blind crossover clinical trial, those women receiving 80 mg of isoflavones daily (45 mg genistein) demonstrated a 26% improvement in arterial wall elasticity compared with the placebo group. Arterial compliance was improved to about the same extent as with HRT (Nestel, Pomeroy, et al., 1997; Nestel, Yamashita, et al., 1997). Low SHBG is also a risk factor for CHD mortality in women (Lapidus et al., 1990). Thus, any compound that raises the SHBG level would have a beneficial effect for heart disease risk.

Phytoestrogens have been demonstrated to have hypocholesterolemic effects in both animal (Sharma, 1979) and human studies. In patients with type II hyperlipoproteinemia, a 14% decrease in serum cholesterol was achieved with a 2-week treatment with a soybean protein diet that included phytoestrogens, and a 21% decrease occurred after 3 weeks (Sirtori, Agradi, Conto, Mantero, & Gatti, 1977). In the same patients, the standard low lipid-low cholesterol diet was ineffective in reducing serum cholesterol.

Phytoestrogens also have a beneficial effect on bone mineral density (Ho, Bacon, Harris, Looker, & Magi, 1993; Kao & P'eng, 1995). Studies focusing on a synthetic but structurally similar compound, ipriflavone (synthetic 7-isopropoxy-isoflavone), also provide evidence that genistein exerts a bone protective effect. In vitro studies have shown a direct inhibitory effect of ipriflavone on bone resorption and on the growth and function of rat osteoblast-like cells (Benvenuti et al., 1991). Short-term clinical trials using small samples of participants have shown that ipriflavone prevents the decline of bone density in older women as well as in bilaterally oophorectomized women (Agnusdei et al., 1989; Agnusdei et al., 1992; Gambacciani et al., 1993). Ho et al. (1993) conducted a small 2-year clinical trial of ipriflavone in healthy, relatively young (aged 50-60) postmenopausal women and found that bone mineral density of the spine decreased significantly for women in the placebo group ($n = 18$) but not in the treatment group ($n = 17$).

Tea as a nonnutrient antioxidant beverage source offers substantial benefit as an alternative to coffee or other caffeinated beverages that have been investigated as a risk factor for bone health (Ferrini & Barrett-Connor, 1996;

Johnell et al., 1995; Lloyd, Rollings, Eggli, Kieselhorst, & Chinchilli, 1997). Green tea consumption, a staple of the Asian diet, has been found to be a protective factor against osteoporosis (Kao & P'eng, 1995). The incidence of osteoporosis-related fractures in Asia is lower there than in most Western communities.

Polyphenols. The polyphenols, a category of nonnutrient antioxidants, occur widely in edible plant material but are especially abundant in green and black tea (Dreosti, 1996). Tea consumption has been most widely studied for its effects on the prevention of cancer (Goldbaum, Hertog, Brants, van Poppel, & van den Brandt, 1996; Huang et al., 1997; Kohlmeier, Weterings, Steck, & Kok, 1997). One recent study focused specifically on postmenopausal women (Zheng et al., 1996).

Several other investigations have suggested that drinking tea provides a degree of protection against cardiovascular disease. Ishikawa et al. (1997) investigated the effect of the intake of five cups of green tea each day on the lipid profile of healthy male volunteers. Biochemical analyses indicated a greater effect on inhibition of oxidation of LDL-C among the tea drinkers, although detectable blood levels of LDL were not significantly different between the tea drinkers and their controls after 4 weeks of study.

Major questions remain about the general advantages of estrogen replacement, time of initiation, and duration of therapy among elderly women. Nevertheless, the weight of the currently available evidence would seem to support the conclusion that HRT improves the atherogenic profile and cognitive functioning of many elderly women, whether it is initiated at menopause or much later. Estrogen will lower the chances of death and disability from cardiovascular disease and osteoporosis. However, for those women unable or unwilling to take HRT, nutritional alternatives directed toward the reduction of cardiovascular risk and osteoporosis are available. Table 4.6 describes dietary sources of phytoestrogens.

PSYCHOSOCIAL HEALTH-PROMOTING INTERVENTIONS

Treatment of Depression

Well-accepted, standardized methods for evaluating depressive symptoms and disorders in older adults have been developed. Criteria for evaluation of depressive symptoms in older people have been established by the American Psychiatric Association (1994) and include key symptoms such as

TABLE 4.6 Dietary Sources of Phytoestrogens

Category	Dietary Source	Specific Foods	Benefits
Isoflavone	Legumes	Soybeans, lentils, kidney and lima beans (Axelson, Sjovall, & Gustafsson, 1994; Knight & Eden, 1995; Price & Fenwick, 1985)	Increased bone mineral density (Kao & P'eng, 1995); increased sex hormone-binding globulin (Lapidus, Lindstredt, Lundberg, Bengston, & Gredmark, 1986); increased arterial wall elasticity (Nestel, Yamashita, et al., 1997); decreases menopausal symptoms (Murkies et al., 1998); reduction of breast cancer (Adlercreutz, 1990)
	Soybean	Tofu, soy milk, soy flour (Dwyer et al., 1994; Messina, 1994)	
Lignans	Whole grain cereal	Rye, brans, oats, rice, barley, wheat, wheat germ	
	Fruits, vegetables, seeds	Linseed, onion, garlic, carrots, pears, cherries, apples, olive oil	

loss of pleasure in daily activities, weight loss, insomnia, fatigue, feelings of worthlessness, diminished ability to think or concentrate, and recurrent thoughts of death. Signs and symptoms of depression may include expressions of sadness, tearfulness, and behavior consistent with increasing dependency (Blazer, 1993; Robinson, 1998).

Effective treatment approaches for depression have been developed, including both pharmaceutical and psychotherapeutic approaches (Robinson, 1998). However, little is known about what combination of pharmacological therapies and psychotherapies are most effective for treating anxiety disorders in older adults. Pharmacologic therapy has been noted as effective in treating depression in older people. Tricyclic antidepressants such as imipramine and doxepin are frequently used for depression in older people. However, tricyclic antidepressants are associated with frequent adverse effects. Thus, attention must be given to drug sensitivity in older people and the need for appropriate dosage. Side effects may include confusion, urinary retention, constipation, tachycardia, and orthostatic hypotension. New classes of tricyclic secondary amines, such as nortriptyline, protriptyline, and desipramine, have fewer side effects than do traditional tricyclics. Tricyclics, trazodone, and fluoxetine also have been successful in treating depression in older adults. Serotonic reuptake inhibitors appear to be effective in treating depression in older people and are noted to be less toxic than the tricyclic antidepressants, but they may not be effective in treating insomnia and anxiety. Side effects may include nausea.

Treatment of depression in older people requires attention to the life patterns and meaning of the individual. Therapy includes building on the worthwhile and meaningful activities of the elderly person, and encouraging the development of relationships with others. It is useful to consider depression in response to the many changes and losses associated with aging in light of the meaning that specific age-related changes have for sense of competence, mastery, ability to adapt to an often challenging environment, and sense of the self (Buckwalter, 1990; Wolfe, Morrow, & Fredrickson, 1996). For many elderly, changes in aspects of physical function involve the loss of valued abilities or personally defining characteristics. In developing therapeutic interventions, it is important to understand the meaning of a particular age-related change for the individual in terms of lifelong patterns of activity, behavior, interests, and personality. Within this context, suggestions can be made to help the individual by adapting coping strategies and other cognitive interventions for reducing stress, including problem-focused coping and problem solving (Blazer, 1993; Buckwalter, 1990).

Continued research is needed to identify the optimal pharmacological and psychological aspects of therapy for treatment of diverse groups of depressed older adults. Therapeutic approaches for the management of elderly individuals with combinations of cognitive, communication, and depressive disorders should be explored. Furthermore, clinical trials and observational studies are needed to identify optimal components of therapy for the very old, older adults from minority or underserved communities, and older adults with a combination of physical illness and depression (Buckwalter, 1990).

Social Network Function and Support

Social contacts and supportive networks are essential to the health of older people. The extent of social networks and support available within the elderly community appears to be related to a number of physical and psychological health outcomes, including functional status, ability to care for oneself, well-being, and quality of life (Binstock, 1997).

A support system has been characterized as an enduring pattern of attachment among individuals and groups that assists older people in managing life's challenges, difficulties, and transitions. Support systems provide guidance in managing short- and long-term problems, offering information and tangible assistance, and promoting a sense of control. Social support may be received from a number of sources, including family, friends, neighbors, church members, and community and voluntary organizations. Social isolation occurs due to a disruption in linkages to a supportive network and may both negatively affect health and promote feelings of vulnerability (Weiss, 1989).

Support networks function in a variety of ways. Supportive relationships have been identified as key in helping older people to maintain physical and psychological health, maintain self-concept, and obtain material aid. Social factors play a dominant role in influencing individual goals, strategies, and opportunities for health promotion. Social support from family and friends has been consistently and positively related to healthy behaviors (Riegel, 1989). Family members, friends, and church members are part of the social context that can affect both the health and sense of well-being of older people. Through integration into a social network, people may experience greater positive affect and higher self-esteem or may feel more in control of behavioral and environmental changes. A growing number of studies show an increased risk of mortality related to lack of social support among older people (Boult, Kane, Louis, Boult, & McCaffrey, 1994; Seeman, Kaplan, Knudsen, Cohen, & Guralnik, 1987; Seeman et al., 1993; Seeman & Syme, 1987; Sugisawa, Liang, & Liu, 1994). In one study, a 30% increased risk of mortality was found among those who had little contact with friends or relatives and little participation in church groups (Seeman et al., 1987). Analyses of mortality data from participants in the Longitudinal Study on Aging showed that low levels of social contact were associated with an increased risk of death (Boult et al., 1994; Steinbach, 1992).

Social network function and support also have been related in a number of studies to functional status in older people. Lack of social contact has been consistently associated with risk of dependency and reduced level of function (Boult et al., 1994; Kaplan et al., 1987, 1993). Camacho, Strawbridge, Cohen, and Kaplan (1993) found that for a group of elders over the age of 80, functional status was better in those who had sustained social relationships over the previous 20 years. Magaziner, Simonsick, Kashner, Hebel, and Kenzora (1990) and Boult et al. (1994) found that higher levels of social contact were associated with improved walking ability and less physical dependence among hip fracture patients.

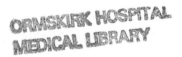

CHAPTER 5

Prevention and Screening

CANCER SCREENING

Following heart disease, cancer is the leading cause of death in older people. Fifty percent of all documented cancer cases occur in 11% of the population over age 65 (Parker, Tong, Bolden, & Wingo, 1996). Among women, one half who develop breast or oral cancer are over age 65; in men, 80% of all cancer of the prostate occurs in older people (Parker et al., 1996). Early detection of cancer is an important clinical strategy in the health promotion efforts of older people, augmenting efforts to reduce morbidity and mortality in this group.

As with other measures to enhance health promotion efforts, there are disparate uses of cancer screening interventions among the poor and minority groups (Mandelblatt, Traxler, Lakin, Kanetsky, & Kao, 1993; Mandelblatt, Traxler, Lakin, Kanetsky, Thomas, et al., 1993). In women, it was shown that education less than 12 years and older than 65 years of age were the most significant explanatory variables in the use of breast exam, cervical screening, and mammography (Mandelblatt, Traxler, Lakin, Kanetsky, & Kao, 1993; Mandelblatt, Traxler, Lakin, Kanetsky, Thomas, et al., 1993).

In women, cancer of the breast represents 45% of all new cases of the disease. Fifty percent of all deaths due to breast cancer are in women over the age of 65 (Mandelblatt, Traxler, Lakin, Kanetsky, & Kao, 1993). Increasing age is the leading risk factor for the disease. Screening for breast cancer includes the breast self-exam, the clinical breast exam, and mammography. Most authorities agree that with the high incidence of breast cancer in older people and with the efficacy of screening, there is no question that screening for breast cancer can save lives (Parker et al., 1996).

The breast self-exam should be performed, following instruction by the clinician, at a designated time every month. The clinical breast examination by a skilled provider should be obtained annually; the same is true of mammography. This preventive screening by the patient and provider is a lifetime requirement and commitment to the preventive health care of the elderly woman.

The incidence of cervical cancer increases with age and continues to be a significant cause of mortality in women. Each year, 27% of new cases and 41% of deaths from cervical cancer occur in elderly women (Mandelblatt, Traxler, Lakin, Kanetsky, & Kao, 1993). The gold standard for screening for cervical cancer is the Papanicolaou (PAP) test. Some authorities suggest that routine PAP screening does not significantly increase life expectancy in older people and should be discontinued after age 65. Other authors disagree, suggesting that there are an alarming number of women who have never been screened, thus increasing their risk of cervical cancer (Mandelblatt, Traxler, Lakin, Kanetsky, Thomas, et al., 1993).

The most common cancer in men is prostate cancer; it is the second leading cause of death in men with cancer (Boring, Squires, Tong, & Montgomery, 1994). Eighty-one percent of all cases of prostate cancer occur in men older than age 65, with half of these occurring in men over age 75. Screening for prostate cancer includes the digital rectal exam, the transrectal ultrasound, and the prostate specific antigen blood test. Conducted annually, these tests, alone or in combination, provide efficacious screening for prostate cancer in the elderly man (Parker et al., 1996).

For those cancers that are amenable to early treatment resulting in increased life expectancy, screening is warranted (Parker et al., 1996). This includes cervical, breast, and prostate cancer screening. Colon cancer, lung cancer, and ovarian cancer screening are not recommended; screening for skin and oral cancers are recommended in high-risk groups (Parker et al., 1996).

The incidence of skin cancer has increased dramatically during the last few decades, with 800,000 to 1.2 million newly diagnosed cases every year (Miller & Weinstock, 1994). One in five individuals in the United States will be diagnosed with skin cancer (Michielutte, Dignan, Sharp, Boxley, & Wells, 1996). The majority of malignancies include nonmelanoma skin cancer, basal cell carcinoma, and squamous cell carcinoma (Federman, Concato, Caralis, Hunkele, & Kirsner, 1997).

Screening for skin cancer demonstrates remarkable efficacy because melanoma has a relatively slow growth phase (Federman et al., 1997). Most adults see their primary health care provider at least every 2 years; most visits include routine examinations (Federman et al., 1997). Thus, the primary care site is the site of choice for skin cancer screening. The American Cancer Society recommends annual skin examinations for all adults 40 years and older (Federman et al., 1997). Some data exist concerning the efficacy of skin cancer screenings, including investigations of the skill of the examiner (Whited, Hall, Russell, Simel, & Horner, 1997). For example, primary care physicians have been shown to include the search for specific malignancies in their examinations, but their examinations may lack sensitivity in general screening (Whited et al., 1997).

For older people, screening and prevention are infrequent health promotion behaviors (Michielutte et al., 1996). The cost of simple preventive measures such as appropriate immunizations and cancer screening are minimal, but they reap major benefits in terms of costly sequelae and quality of life. Health preventive efforts should be a major component of health promotion in older people and the target of interventions directed toward increased frequency of prevention services.

IMMUNE SUPPORT

Immunologic function declines with age, as do most physiologic functions. Concomitant with this decline in immune function is a rise in the incidence of many infections and malignancies with age (Burns & Goodwin, 1997). There is greater morbidity and mortality associated with infections and malignancies associated with common infections in adults over age 65 years. Elderly persons respond less well to protective immunizations against common infections such as influenza and pneumococcal pneumonia. Although immune system alterations are known to be associated with aging and are known to contribute to increased morbidity and mortality in older people, few interventions have been successful in enhancing the immune response of older people.

Immunization refers to the process of inducing or providing immunity artificially by administering a vaccine, toxoid, or antibody-containing preparation. *Active immunization* is defined as the administration of a vaccine or toxoid leading to an immunologic response and the production of specific antibody or antitoxin. *Passive immunization* means that there is provision of temporary immunity by administering preformed antibodies or antitoxin. Specific vaccine indications in adults will vary by lifestyle factors, occupation, or chronic medical conditions. However, in the United States, deaths from vaccine-preventable diseases occur predominantly in adults and particularly in older people. An estimated 50,000 to 70,000 yearly deaths occur among adults from pneumococcal infection, influenza, and hepatitis B (Stollerman, 1997). Influenza and pneumonia remain the fifth-leading cause of death in older people.

Influenza, pneumococcal, and tetanus-diphtheria vaccines are the only vaccines specifically recommended for routine use in older people by the Immunization Advisory Committee of the Centers for Disease Control (CDC) and by the American College of Physicians Task Force on Adult Immunizations. In addition, the CDC now emphasizes the importance of appropriately vaccinating adults against diphtheria, hepatitis B, influenza, measles, mumps, pneumococcal disease, rubella, tetanus, and varicella. Despite some measurable degree of immune senescence with normative aging, vaccine-induced immune responses are still effective in older people who do not suffer from serious morbid or iatrogenic immune compromises. The primary care of all elderly patients should include proper immunizations with at least three vaccines and others, particularly hepatitis B, wherever risk of exposure warrants such protection. The Task Force on Adult Immunization has recommended that age 50 be established as a time for review of preventive health measures, with special emphasis on evaluating risk factors that would include the need for giving pneumococcal vaccine and initiating annual influenza immunization.

Pneumococcal Vaccine

There are an estimated 150,000 to 570,000 cases of pneumococcal pneumonia per year, with an estimated mortality of 5%. Despite appropriate antimicrobial therapy, the mortality rates for pneumonia have not improved greatly in recent decades. The rising frequency and dissemination of strains of multiply antibiotic-resistant pneumococci have made the priority for antipneumococcal immunization very high (Breiman, Butler, Tenover, Elliott, & Facklam, 1994).

Three primary factors influence the efficacy of the vaccine: immune competence, age at the time of infection, and time since vaccination. Efficacy can range from 93% for an immunocompetent person under age 55 who had been vaccinated less than 3 years before to no protection for an immunocompetent person over age 85 more than 5 years after immunization (Shapiro et al., 1991). National organizations including the Immunization Practices Advisory Committee of the CDC recommend pneumococcal vaccination in all persons 65 years of age or older and persons of any age who are at high risk because of conditions such as chronic illness, diabetes mellitus, and organ transplant. Individuals who received pneumococcal vaccine before age 65 years, because of their risk factors, should be considered candidates for reimmunization at age 65, provided at least 6 years have passed since they received the first dose of vaccine. The vaccine offers as much protection against drug-resistant as against sensitive pneumococci (Stollerman, 1997). Most healthy adults develop type-specific antibodies in 2 to 3 weeks, but the titer of antibody protective against each serotype has not been determined. Adverse reactions to the vaccine are minor. Approximately half of those vaccinated will have local soreness. More severe allergic or systemic reactions are seen in fewer than 1% of recipients.

Pneumococcal vaccine should be given as a single intramuscular injection of 0.05 ml. Protective antibodies usually persist for at least 5 to 10 years after immunization in immunocompetent hosts and not as long in less competent hosts. Although the optimal time for revaccination needs to be determined, in those immunocompromised—including those with renal failure, transplant recipients, and patient with HIV infection—revaccination every 5 to 6 years should be considered. There is no evidence that routine revaccination is of benefit in other groups.

Influenza Vaccine

More lives and health care dollars are lost by influenza-related illness than by any other virus-caused disease in the United States. Persons greater than 60 years of age account for about 80% to 90% of excess deaths from influenza. Influenza vaccination is indicated for all persons who are at increased risk of influenza-related complications, such as older people or for those who, if infected, can transfer influenza to older people (Stollerman, 1997). The vaccine has been proven to be both protective and cost-effective.

Influenza vaccines are constituted to provide protection against the influenza virus's two major surface antigens, the neuroaminidases (N1, N2) and the hemagglutinin (H1, H2, H3). Disease from influenza A viruses tends to be more severe than that caused by influenza B viruses. The protection afforded by influenza vaccination is best correlated with the development of serum hemagglutinin antibodies. Viral subtypes undergo yearly antigenic variation that may result in one strain not inducing immunity to related strains of the same subtype. When there is a good match between vaccine and circulating viruses, influenza vaccine is at least 70% effective in preventing hospitalization for pneumonia among elderly living in the community. Among elderly persons in chronic care facilities, influenza vaccine is 50% to 60% effective in preventing hospitalization and pneumonia and 80% effective in preventing death.

The vaccine should be administered intramuscularly in one dose of 0.5 ml during the fall each year. There is little or no improvement in antibody responses when a second dose is given to adults during the same season. Protective antibody titers against influenza infection are achieved about 2 weeks after vaccination and begin to decline after 4 to 6 months. Influenza vaccine may be given along with pneumoccal vaccine but at separate sites. Soreness at the injection site disappearing at 1 to 2 days is the most common adverse reaction. Occasionally fever, malaise, and myalgia may occur, but these last no more than 1 to 2 days. Severe hypersensitivity reactions are very rare. Although influenza vaccination can alter the hepatic clearance of drugs, including warfarin, theophylline, and phenytoin, none of these effects is clinically significant. Anaphylactic hypersensitivity to eggs has been considered a contraindication because of the egg-grown origin of the vaccine.

Influenza vaccine must be given annually, both because of a short-lived protective response and because of variation in prevalent infecting strains each year. It must be given each year within a few months of the onset of the influenza winter season of December to March.

Tetanus and Diphtheria

Older adults who have not received a primary series of immunizations are the major population at risk for tetanus and diphtheria. Although rare, 60% of cases of tetanus occur in people over 60 years of age, and the case fatality is approximately 50% in this population (Stollerman, 1997). The risk for tetanus and its associated mortality increases with age, as protective antitoxin levels decline and skin wounds and lesions increase. Twenty percent of tetanus cases have been associated with chronic wounds or abscesses, and 55% of these occurred in individuals age 60 or older.

Tetanus-diphtheria toxoid (Td) is recommended for routine use in adults. Three intramuscular doses complete a primary series. A complete primary series consists of two doses of 0.5 ml each intramuscularly, given at least 4 weeks apart, followed by a third reinforcing dose 0.5 ml 6 to 12 months later. Thereafter, a booster dose of 0.5 ml should be given every 10 years, unless the individual suffers a tetanus-prone wound. Tetanus boosting for older persons has been recommended because older persons have the lowest levels of immunity (less than 30% for those older than age 70); although there have been fewer than 100 cases annually nationwide for years, the majority of cases and deaths occur among older adults. Special emphasis should be given to assure that all adults have completed a primary immunization series with Td, followed by a single midlife booster of Td at age 50 for individuals who have completed the full primary series, including the young adult booster. Approximately half of adults age 60 or older have protective titers of circulating antitoxin. Adult susceptibility to diphtheria reflects reduced lifetime exposure to C. diphtheriae and failure to administer a primary series of the vaccine and a booster each decade.

The Td vaccine is among the most immunogenic and effective of all those available. All adults should be actively immunized against both diseases. The requirement for booster injections every 10 years, however, makes older people vulnerable to the consequences of poor primary health care, which may result in the neglect of the maintenance of this immunity. A booster dose given as long as 25 to 30 years after a primary series produces rapid and significant immune response to both toxoids. Tetanus prophylaxis in routine management of clean, minor wounds requires administration of Td only to update primary series. All other wounds should be treated with Td if more than 5 years have passed since the last booster. Tetanus immune globulin is recommended for other than clean, minor wounds when the individual has received fewer than three Td doses in the past or if the history of past tetanus immunization is unknown.

Minor side effects to Td are common, with about 60% reporting at least one reaction. Side effects may include sore arm, swelling at the site of injection, and itching. A history of neurologic symptoms or severe hypersensitivity reaction following a previous Td dose is a contraindication to primary immunization or additional boosters.

Other Vaccines

In addition to giving vaccines that are routinely recommended, physicians should ask all older adults about their lifestyles, occupations, and special circumstances, such as impending travel, that may prompt consideration of other vaccines. Screening geriatric patients routinely for their immunization needs offers the opportunity to note those who may still be at special risk by occupation, household, and institutional environment and lifestyle, and thereby eligible for hepatitis B vaccine.

New vaccines are becoming available that may be of importance to elderly patients. Hepatitis A vaccine can be expected to replace immunoglobulin to prevent hepatitis A and may be particularly relevant to elderly travelers to areas where the risk of hepatitis is high.

CHAPTER 6

Directions for Research and Intervention

The challenge for health promotion and disease prevention requires that researchers and clinicians explore new ways to address the problem of health promotion in older people. The most salient of lifestyle behaviors that affect health outcomes in primary, secondary, and tertiary promotion and prevention efforts have been presented in this volume. However, there are many considerations extant in developing targeted interventions to reduce risk and promote healthy behaviors. Little attention has been paid to how to promote behaviors that decrease use of medical services, maintain health, and reduce disability into old age. Research on how to promote behaviors that are effective in preventing and managing chronic illness is greatly needed. Primary care practitioners must begin to explore the most effective techniques for promoting sustained risk reducing health behaviors in older adults. It is currently not known what may be the most effective target for intervention strategies. Should interventions occur at the level of the individual, the work force, or the community? More work must be done on the cultural, socioeconomic, and societal conditions under which individuals become motivated to change health behaviors; the roles of social support systems in adopting and maintaining changes; and the most effective settings and types of interventions that result in sustained health-promoting behaviors. Due to the complexity of efforts directed toward health promotion in older people, four considerations are offered the clinician in developing targeted interventions:

1. The importance of thorough and appropriate assessments
2. The importance of lifestyle changes in achieving health promotion and disease prevention outcomes
3. The importance of culturally sensitive efforts
4. The importance of theory-based interventions

THE IMPORTANCE OF THOROUGH AND APPROPRIATE ASSESSMENTS

The process and content of interventions for the older individual is much different than those addressed in younger individuals. The window of opportunity for behavior change and screening efforts in older people is quite narrow. The physical and physiological changes accompanying aging leaves, for some individuals, little opportunity for significant changes in health outcomes following health behavior changes. In addition, there is little empirical evidence as to the efficacy of some targeted interventions, such as dietary intake alterations in the reduction of unfavorable lipids. Thus, for each intervention, each prescription for nutritional change, clinical assessments of the older individual's functional capabilities must be made. Assessment of his or her environment in terms of safety, resources, and social support to sustain behavioral changes needs to be considered.

THE IMPORTANCE OF LIFESTYLE CHANGES IN ACHIEVING HEALTHY OUTCOMES

This volume synthesizes the empirical evidence that the major lifestyle health promotion efforts of cigarette smoking cessation, physical activity, and appropriate nutritional intake have direct relation to the reduced risk of disease, the secondary prevention of adverse sequelae, and improved quality of life. As stated previously, the window of opportunity in the older individual may be more narrow than that of a younger person, but the evidence remains that there are large risk reduction gains achieved with small changes in, for example, systolic blood pressure reduction and use of hormone replacement therapy. Older individuals benefit from screening efforts. For example, survival data on breast cancer shows that older persons have relative survival rates as high as those among many younger age groups.

THE IMPORTANCE OF CULTURALLY SENSITIVE HEALTH PROMOTION EFFORTS

The rapid pace of growth in the numbers and proportions of older individuals with diverse ethnic origins directs the necessity for targeting interventions toward an appropriate cultural context. In later years of life, the minority elderly, more than other groups, face old age with a lifetime of racial discrimination, marginal living conditions, and quality of life inequities. For the older immigrant individual, the lack of resources and comfort with the mainstream society hamper health promotion efforts. Investigators who choose to examine health issues in older people, many of whom are disadvantaged, need to resist the assumption that strategies that have been successful in certain segments of the population are appropriate for those older individuals who lack the resources to overcome the social and economic bias against positive health behaviors. Each intervention should be designed with the target ethnic or racial group considered and include individual variations in communication, family and kinship, and resources.

THE IMPORTANCE OF THEORY-BASED INTERVENTIONS

The value of individual models of health behavior is without question. However, their relevance as a guide for intervention in the socially and economically disadvantaged is questionable. We must move beyond a high-risk approach to disease management to include those determinants of health-related behavior change that are embedded in the relationships that tie individuals to organizations, neighborhoods, families, and friends in their community.

Conceptual models of health are needed to encourage policymakers to devise multifaceted approaches to health promotion (Collins, 1995). New ways of conceptualizing the determinants of health are needed to promote an awareness of the full spectrum of factors that can contribute to health or its absence. For community programs to be successful, efforts are needed to promote the adoption of the health promotion program throughout systems and neighboring communities. Many health promotion programs, both individual and community-based, have focused mainly on promotional strategies for immediate results without attention to widespread and long-term change (Murdaugh & Vanderboom, 1997).

Efforts must be made to develop and apply motivational theories to community-based interventions for the creation of competent communities.

The achievement of these goals for older people might best occur through a combination of community development and social action strategies. Both approaches involve increased participation in decision making by older people in the community. Any program designed to enhance empowerment and community competence in older people must begin with an understanding of the environmental context and experiences of older individuals as community members (i.e., the person-environment fit). Three factors that are thought to differentiate more competent from less competent communities include (a) the power to generate alternatives and opportunities, (b) knowledge of where and how to obtain resources, and (c) self-esteem in the form of optimism and motivation (Iscoe, 1974).

Older individuals as members of families and communities can be empowered to establish their own health priorities and be involved in the selection of treatments as well as the development and implementation of relevant programs to address the social problem of disease prevention and health promotion. Only after understanding the context for health promotion activities is it appropriate to design and conduct intervention studies.

Aspects of empowerment for older people must include strategies designed to build on existing individual and community strengths. The generation of alternatives and opportunities for community-based change might focus initially on one risk area of primary concern for women, such as leisure-time activity or safety needs. Alternatives and opportunities may be explored through an open communication forum for identifying potential risk factors, exploring how and why these factors occur, and identifying mechanisms for risk reduction. For example, the older person may identify stress due to social isolation as a barrier to health promotion efforts. One method to reduce this isolation may be to create mechanisms for social support. Older individuals in the community may form formal or informal support groups to share their concerns and identify potential solutions. Support groups may provide tangible support in the form of shared tasks or take a recreational focus, such as the creation of groups that commit to exercising together.

Supportive communication among older people also provides an opportunity to share experiences and knowledge about the availability of resources and how to access needed resources. Support groups may serve as a force to create educational opportunities in the community, including health information and screening. Problem solving and the identification of needed resources also may serve to enhance member self-esteem and motivation in risk modification. Members may work together to identify strengths and resources. The development of relevant role models for risk management in a supportive environment may enhance personal efficacy and create the potential for environmental and individual change.

Individual, community, and social changes are necessary to overcome significant risk factors for health risk in older people, including traditional risk factors, inadequate financial resources, environmental stresses, lack of access to health care, and social isolation. We must begin to explore with older people the potential solutions to individual, community, and systemwide problems to better understand "risk" in a larger context and to develop more effective and relevant community interventions.

References

Aday, L. A. (1993). *At risk in America: The health and health care needs of vulnerable populations in the United States.* San Francisco: Jossey-Bass.

Adlercreutz, H. (1990). Western diet and Western diseases: Some hormonal and biochemical mechanisms and associations. *Scandinavian Journal of Clinical Laboratory Investigation, 50*(Suppl. 20), 3-23.

Adlercreutz, H., Bannwart, C., Wahala, K., Makela, T., Brunow, G., Hase, T., Arosemena, P. J., Kellis, J. T., Jr., & Vickery, L. E. (1993) Inhibition of human aromatase by mammalian lignans and isoflavonoid phytoestrogens. *Journal of Steroid Biochemistry & Molecular Biology, 44,* 147-153.

Adlercreutz, H., Hockerstedt, K., Bannwart, C., Bloigu, S., Hamalainen, E., Fotsis, T., & Ollus, A. (1987). Effect of dietary components including lignans and phytoestrogens on enterhepatic circulation and liver metabolism of estrogens and sex hormone binding globulin. *Journal of Steroid Biochemistry, 27,* 1135-1144.

Adlercreutz, H., Honjo, H., Higashi, A., Fotsis, T., Hamalainen, E., Hasegawa, T., & Okada, H. (1991). Urinary excretion of lignans and isoflavonoid phytoestrogens in Japanese men and women consuming a traditional Japanese diet. *American Journal of Clinical Nutrition, 54,* 1093-1100.

Agnee, E. (1986). *A portrait of older minorities: American Association of Retired Persons.* Washington, DC: Minority Affairs Initiative.

Agnusdei, D., Camporeale, A., Gonnelli, S., Gennari, C., Baroni, M. C., & Passeri, M. (1992). Short-term treatment of Paget's disease of bone with ipriflavone. *Bone & Mineral, 19*(Suppl. 1), 35-42

Agnusdei, D., Zacchei, F., Bigazzi, S., Cepollaro, C., Nardi, P., Montagnani, M., & Gennari, C. (1989). Metabolic and clinical effects of ipriflavone in established post-menopausal osteoporosis. *Drugs Experimental and Clinical Research, 15,* 97-104.

Airhihenbuwa, C. O., Kumanyika, S., Agurs, T. D., & Lowe, A. (1995). Perceptions and beliefs about exercise, rest, and health among African-Americans. *American Journal of Health Promotion, 9,* 426-429.

Ajzen, I., & Fishbein, M. (1980). *Understanding attitudes and predicting social behavior.* Englewood Cliffs, NJ: Prentice Hall.

Albert, C. M., Hennekens, C. H., O'Donnell, C. J., Ajani, U. A., Carey, V. J., Willett, W. C., Ruskin, J. N., & Manson, J. E. (1998). Fish consumption and risk of sudden cardiac death. *Journal of the American Medical Association, 279,* 23-28.

Albert, M. S. (1994). Cognition and aging. In W. R. Hazzard, E. L. Bierman, I. P. Blass, et al. (Eds.), *Principles of geriatric medicine and gerontolgy* (3rd ed., pp. 1013-1020). New York: McGraw-Hill.

Allman, R. (1989). Pressure sores among the elderly. *New England Journal of Medicine, 320,* 850-853.

Alpha-Tocopherol, Beta Carotene Cancer Prevention Study Group. (1994). The effect of vitamin E and beta carotene on the incidence of lung cancer and other cancers in male smokers. *New England Journal of Medicine, 330,* 1029-1035.

American Diabetes Association. (1989). Role of cardiovascular risk factors in prevention and treatment of microvascular disease in diabetes. *Diabetes Care, 12,* 573-579.

American Heart Association. (1998). *Heart and stroke facts statistics.* Dallas, TX: Author.

American Psychiatric Association. (1994). *Diagnostic and statistical manual of mental disorders* (4th ed.). Washington, DC: Author.

Andersen, R. E., Wadden, T. A., Bartlett, S. J., Vogt, R. A., & Weinstock, R. S. (1995). Relation of weight loss to changes in serum lipids and lipoproteins in obese women. *American Journal of Clinical Nutrition, 62,* 350-357.

Anderson, K. M., & Kannel, W. B. (1992). Obesity and disease. In B. Bjorntorp & B. N. Brodoff (Eds.), *Obesity* (pp. 465-473). Philadelphia: J. B. Lippincott.

Aneshensel, C. S., & Pearlin, L. I. (1987). Structural contexts of differences in stress. In R. C. Barnett, G. K. Baruch, & L. Biener (Eds.), *Gender and stress* (pp. 75-95). New York: Free Press.

Aniansson, A., & Gustafsson, E. (1981). Physical training in elderly men with special reference to quadriceps muscle strength and morphology. *Clinical Physiology, 1,* 87-98.

Anthony, J. C., & Aboraya, A. (1992). The epidemiology of selected mental disorders in later life. In J. E. Birren, R. B. Sloane, & G. D. Cohen (Eds.), *Handbook of mental health and aging* (2nd ed., pp. 27-73). San Diego, CA: Academic Press.

Ashley, F. W., & Kannel, W. B. (1974). Relationship to weight change in atherogenic traits: The Framingham study. *Journal of Chronic Disease, 27,* 103-114.

Assaf, A. R., Banspach, S. W., & Laster, T. M. (1987). The Pawtucket Heart Health Program: Evaluation strategies. *Rhode Island Medical Journal, 70,* 546-641.

Avis, N. E., Brambilla, D., McKinaly, S. M., & Vass, K. (1994). A longitudinal analysis of the association between menopause and depression. Results from the Massachusetts Women's Health Study. *Annals of Epidemiology, 4,* 214-220.

Axelson, M., Sjovall, J., & Gustafsson, B. E. (1994). Soya—A dietary source of the nonsteroidal estrogen equol in man and animals. *Journal of Endocrinology, 102,* 49-56.

Bailey, E. J. (1987). Sociocultural factors and health care-seeking behavior among black Americans. *Journal of the National Medical Association, 79,* 389-392.

Baker, G. T., & Martin, G. R. (1997). Molecular biologic factors in aging: The origins, causes, and presentation of senescence. In C. K. Cassel, H. J. Cohen, E. B. Larson, D. E. Meier, N. M. Resnick, L. Z. Rubenstein, & L. B. Sorensen (Eds.), *Geriatric medicine* (3rd ed., pp. 3-28). New York: Springer.

Balin, A. K., & Allen, R. G. (1986). Mechanisms of biologic aging. *Dermatology Clinic, 4,* 347-358.

Ballor, D. L., & Poehlman, E. T. (1994). Exercise-training enhances fat-free mass preservation during diet-induced weight loss: A meta-analytical finding. *International Journal of Obesity and Related Metabolic Disorder, 18*(1), 35-40.

Balsam, A. L., & Bottum, C. L. (1997). Understanding the aging and public health networks. In T. Hickey, M. A. Speers, & T. R. Prohaska (Eds.), *Public health and aging* (pp. 17-36). Baltimore: Johns Hopkins University Press.

Bandura, A. (1986). *Social foundations of thought and action.* Englewood Cliffs, NJ: Prentice Hall.

Bandura, A. (1997). *Self-Efficacy: The exercise of control.* New York: Freeman.

Baranowski, T. (1995). A center-based program for exercise change among Black-American families. *Health Education Quarterly, 17*(2), 179-196.

Barrett-Connor, E., & Bush, T. L. (1991). Estrogen and coronary heart disease in women. *Journal of the American Medical Association, 265,* 1861-1867.

Barrett-Connor, E., & Miller, V. (1993). Estrogens, lipids, and heart disease. *Clinics in Geriatric Medicine, 9*(1), 57-67.

Becker, D. M., Windsor, R., Ockene, J. K., Berman, B., Best, J. A., Cummings, K. M., Glantz, S., Haynes, S., Henningfield, J., Novotry, T. E., Orleans, C. T., & Prochas, J. O. (1993). AHA prevention conference III behavior change and compliance: Keys to improving cardiovascular health, January 15-17, 1993, Monterey, California: Setting the policy, advocation, research agenda to reduce tobacco use: Workshop I. *Circulation, 88,* 1381-1386.

Belisle, M., Roskies, E., & Levesque, J. M. (1987). Improving adherence to physical activity. *Health Psychology, 6*(2), 159-172.

Benvenuti, S., Tanini, A., Frediani, U., Bianchi, S., Masi, L., Casano, R., Bufalino, L., Serio, M., & Brandi, M. L. (1991). Effects of inpriflavone and its metabolities on a clonal esteoblastic cell line. *Journal of Bone and Mineral Research, 6,* 987-996.

Bergman, E. A., & Boyungs, J. C. (1991). Indoor walking program increases lean body composition in older women. *Journal of the American Dietetic Association, 91,* 1433-1435.

Berkman, L. F., & Seeman, T. (1986). The influence of social relationships on aging and the development of cardiovascular disease—A review. *Postgraduate Medical Journal, 62,* 805-807.

Bertram, J. S., & Bortkiewicz, H. (1995). Dietary carotenoids inhibit neoplastic transformation and module gene expression in mouse and humans. *American Journal of Clinical Nutrition, 62*(Suppl. 6), 1327-1336.

Binstock, R. H. (1997). Issues of resource allocation in an aging society. In T. Hickey, M. A. Speers, & T. R. Prohaska (Eds.), *Public health and aging* (pp. 54-72). Baltimore: Johns Hopkins University Press.

Bjorntorp, P. (1990). "Portal" adipose tissue as a generator of risk factors for cardiovascular disease and diabetes. *Arteriosclerosis, 10,* 493-496.

Bjorntorp, P. (1992). Regional obesity. In P. Bjorntorp & B. N. Brodoff (Eds.), *Obesity* (pp. 579-586). Philadelphia: J. B. Lippincott.

Blair, S. N., Kohl, H. W., & Gordon, N. F. (1992). How much physical activity is good for health? *Annual Review of Public Health, 13,* 99-126.

Blair, S. N., Kohl, H. W., Paffenbarger, R. S., Clark, D. G., Cooper, K. H., & Gibbons, L. W. (1989). Physical fitness and all-cause mortality: A prospective study of healthy men and women. *Journal of the American Medical Association, 262,* 2395-2401.

Blazer, D. (1993). *Depression in late life* (2nd ed.). St Louis, MO: C.V. Mosby.

Blumenthal, J. A., Emery, C. F., Madden, D. J., Coleman, R. E., Riddle, M. W., Schniebolk, S., Cobb, F. R., Sullivan, M. J., & Higginbotham, M. B. (1991). Effects of exercise training on cardiorespiratory function in men and women older than 60 years of age. *American Journal of Cardiology, 67,* 633-639.

Bogden, J. D., Oleske, J. M., Munves, E. M., Lavenhar, M. A., Bruening, K. S., Kemp, F. W., Holding, K. J., Denny, T. N., & Louria, D. B. (1987). Zinc and immunocompetence in the elderly: Baseline data on zinc nutriture and immunity in unsupplemented subjects. *American Journal of Clinical Nutrition, 46*(1), 101-109.

Bootzin, R. R., Quan, S. F., Bamford, C. R., & Wyatt, J. K. (1995). Sleep disorders. *Comprehensive Therapy, 21,* 401-406.

Borchelt, M., & Horgas, A. L. (1994). Screening an elderly population for verifiable adverse drug reactions: Methodological approach and initial data of the Berlin Aging Study (BASE). *Annals of the New York Academy of Sciences, 717,* 270-281.

Borg, G. A. V. (1982). Psychophysical bases of perceived exertion. *Medicine and Science in Sports and Exercise, 14,* 377-381.

Boring, C. C., Squires, T. S., Tong, T., & Montgomery, S. (1994). Cancer statistics, 1994. *CA: A Cancer Journal for Clinicians, 44*(1), 7-26

Bortz, W. M. (1996). Human aging—Normal and abnormal. In D. W. Jahnigen & R. W. Schrier (Eds.), *Geriatric medicine* (2nd ed., pp. 3-17). Cambridge, MA: Blackwell.

Boult, C., Kane, R., Louis, T., Boult, L., & McCaffrey, D. (1994). Chronic conditions that lead to functional limitation in the elderly. *Journal of Gerontology, 49*(1), M28-M36.

Boushey, C. J., Beresford, S. A., Omenn, G. S., & Motulsky, A. G. (1995). A quantitative assessment of plasma homocysteine as a risk factor for vascular disease. Probable benefits of increasing folic acid intakes. *Journal of the American Medical Association, 274,* 1049-1057.

Branch, L. G., Katz, S., Kneipman, K., & Papsidero, J. (1984). A prospective study of functional status among community elders. *American Journal of Public Health, 74,* 266-268.

Branch, L. G., Walker, L. A., Wetle, T. T., DuBeau, C. E., & Resnick, N. M. (1994). Urinary incontinence knowledge among community dwelling people 65 years of age and older. *Journal of the American Geriatric Society, 42,* 1257-1262.

Bray, G. A. (1987). Overweight is risking fate: Definition, classification, prevalence, and risks. *Annals of the New York Academy of Sciences, 499,* 14-28.

Breder, C. D., Dinarello, C. A., & Saper, C. B. (1988). Interleukin-1 immunoreactive innervation of the human hypothalamus. *Science, 240,* 321-324.

Breen, N., & Figueroa, J. B. (1996). Stage of breast and cervical cancer diagnosis in disadvantaged neighborhoods: A prevention policy perspective. *American Journal of Preventive Medicine, 12,* 319-326.

Breiman, R. F., Butler, J. C., Tenover, F. C., Elliott, J. A., & Facklam, R. R. (1994). Emergence of drug-resistant pneumococcal infections in the United States. *Journal of the American Medical Association, 271,* 1831-1835.

Brody, J. A., Brock, D. B., & Williams, T. F. (1987). Trends in the health of the elderly population. *Annual Review of Public Health, 8,* 211-234.

Brown, A. B., McCartney, N., & Sale, D. G. (1990). Positive adaptations to weight-lifting training in the elderly. *Journal of Applied Physiology, 69,* 1725-1733.

Brummel-Smith, K. (1998). Polypharmacy and the elderly patient. *Archives of the American Academy of Orthopaedic Surgeons, 2,* 39-44.

Brzezinski, A., Adlercreutz, H., Shaoul, R., Rosler, A., Shmueli, A., Tano, V., & Schenker, J. G. (1997). Short-term effects of phytoestrogen-rich diet on postmenopausal women. *Journal of the North American Menopause Society, 4*(2), 89-94.

Buchkremer, G., Minneker, E., & Block, M. (1991). Smoking-cessation treatment combining transdermal nicotine substitution with behavioral therapy. *Pharmacopsychiatry, 24*(3), 96-102.

Buckwalter, K. C. (1990, July/August). How to unmask depression. *Geriatric Nursing,* 179-181.

Buring, J. E., Hebert, P., Romero, J., Kittross, A., Cook, N., Manson, J., Peto, R., & Hennekens, C. (1995). Migraine and subsequent risk of stroke in the Physicians' Health Study. *Archives of Neurology, 52*(2), 129-134.

Burke, L. B., Jolson, H. M., Goetsch, R. A., & Ahronheim, J. C. (1992). Focus on medication in the elderly. In J. W. Rowe & J. C. Ahronheim (Eds.), *Annual review of gerontology and geriatrics* (Vol. 12, p. 1028). New York: Springer.

Burns, E. A., & Goodwin, J. S. (1997). Changes in immunologic function. In C. K. Cassel, H. J. Cohen, E. B. Larson, D. E. Meier, N. M. Resnick, L. Z. Rubenstein, & L. B. Sorensen (Eds.), *Geriatric medicine* (3rd ed., pp. 585-597). New York: Springer.

Buskirk, E. R. (1985). Health maintenance and longevity: Exercise. In C. E. Finch & E. L. Schneider (Eds.), *Handbook of the biology of aging* (2nd ed., pp. 894-931). New York: Van Nostrand Rienhold.

Camacho, T., Strawbridge, W., Cohen, R., & Kaplan, G. (1993). Functional ability in the oldest old: Cumulative impact of risk factors from the preceding two decades. *Journal of Aging and Health, 5,* 439-454.

Campbell, W. W., Crim, M. C., Dallal, G. E., Young, V. R., & Evans, W. J. (1994). Increased protein requirements in elderly people: New data and retrospective reassessments. *American Journal of Clinical Nutrition, 60,* 501-509.

Campbell, W. W., Crim, M. C., Young, V. R., Joseph, L. J., & Evans, W. J. (1995). Effects of resistance training and dietary protein intake on protein metabolism in older adults. *American Journal of Physiology, 268*(6 Pt. 1), E1143-E1153.

Cardinal, B. J., & Sachs, M. L. (1996). Effects of mail-mediated, stage-matched exercise behavior change strategies on female adults' leisure-time exercise behavior. *Journal of Sports Medicine and Physical Fitness, 36*(2), 100-107.

Carleton, R. A., & Lasater, T. M. (1994). Population intervention to reduce coronary heart disease incidence. In T. Pearson, M. H. Criqui, R. V. Luepker, A. Oberman, & M. Winston (Eds.), *Primer in preventive cardiology* (pp. 285-292). Dallas, TX: American Heart Association.

Carter, W. J. (1991). Macronutrient requirements for elderly persons. In R. Chernoff (Ed.), *Geriatric nutrition* (pp. 11-24). Gaithersburg, MD: Aspen.

Cauley, J. A., Lucas, F. L., Kuller, L. H., Vogt, M. T., Browner, W. S., & Cummings, S. R. (1996). Bone mineral density and risk of breast cancer in older women: The study of osteoporotic fractures. *Journal of the American Medical Association, 276,* 1404-1408.

Census Bureau. (1990). *Poverty in the United States: 1991* (Current Population Reports, no. 75, p. 60). Washington, DC: Government Printing Office.

Chandra, M., Chandra, N., Agrawal, R. K., Ghatak, A., & Pandy, V. C. (1994). The free radical system in ischemic heart disease. *International Journal of Cardiology, 43,* 121-125.

Chandra, R. K. (1990). Nutrition is an important determinant of immunity in old age. *Progress in Clinical Biological Research, 326,* 321-334.

Chandra, R. K. (1997). Graying of the immune system. Can nutrient supplements improve immunity in the elderly? *Journal of the American Medical Association, 277,* 1398-1399.

Charette, S. L., McEvoy, L., Pyka, G., Snow-Harter, C., Guido, D., Wiswell, R. A., & Marcus, R. (1991). Muscle hypertrophy response to resistance training in older women. *Journal of Applied Physiology, 70,* 1912-1916.

Chen, H. C., Ashton-Miller, J. A., Alexander, N. B., & Schultz, A. B. (1994). Effects of age and available response time on ability to step over an obstacle. *Journal of Gerontology, 49*(5), M227-M233.

Chen, M. S., Jr., Kuun, P., Guthrie, R., Li, W., & Zaharlick, A. (1991). Promoting heart health for Southeast Asians: A database for planning interventions. *Public Health Report, 106,* 304-309.

Chernoff, R. (1994). Thirst and fluid requirements. *Nutritional Reviews, 52*(8, Pt. 2), 53-55.

Chernoff, R. (1995). Effects of age on nutrient requirements. *Clinics in Geriatric Medicine, 11,* 641-651.

Chernoff, R., & Lipschitz, D. A. (1985). Aging and nutrition. *Comprehensive Therapy, 11*(8), 29-34.

Chodzko-Zajko, W. J. (1991). Physical fitness, cognitive performance, and aging. *Medicine Science & Sports Exercise, 23,* 868-872.

Chodzko-Zajko, W. J., & Moore, K. A. (1994). Physical fitness and cognitive functioning in aging. *Exercise and Sport Sciences Reviews, 22,* 195-220.

Chow, R., Harrison, J. E., & Notarius, C. (1987). Effect of two randomized exercise programs on bone mass of healthy post menopausal women. *British Medical Journal, 295,* 1141-1144.

Chrischilles, E. A., Segar, E. T., & Wallace, R. B. (1992). Self-reported adverse drug reactions and related resource use: A study of community-dwelling persons 65 years of age and older. *Annals of Internal Medicine, 117,* 634-640.

Clarke, R., Daly, L., Robinson, K., Naughten, E., Cahalane, S., Fowler, B., & Graham, I. (1991). Hyperhomocysteinemia: An independent risk factor for vascular disease. *New England Journal of Medicine, 324,* 1149-1150.

Coalition of Hispanic Health and Human Services Organizations. (1995). Meeting and health promotion needs of Hispanic communities (policy and research, National Coalition of Hispanic Health and Human Services Organizations). *American Journal of Health Promotion, 9,* 300-311.

Cohen, B. B. (1984). A combined approach using meditation-hypnosis and behavioral techniques in the treatment of smoking behavior: Case studies of five stressed patients. *International Journal of Psychosomatics, 31*(1), 33-39.

Cohen, G. (1990). Lessons from longitudinal studies of mentally ill and mentally healthy elderly: A 17 year perspective. In M. Bergener & S. I. Finkel (Eds.), *Clinical and scientific psychogeriatrics* (Vol. 1., pp. 135-148). New York: Springer.

Cohen, S., Lichtenstein, E., Prochaska, J. O., Rossi, J. S., Gritz, E. R., Carr, C. R., Orleans, C. T., Schoenbach, V. J., Biener, L., Abrams, D., DiClemente, C., Curry, S., Marlatt, G. A., Cummings, K. M., Emont, S. L., Giovino, G., & Ossip-Klein, D. (1989). Debunking myths about self-quitting: Evidence from 10 prospective studies of persons who attempt to quit smoking by themselves. *American Psychology, 44,* 1355-1365.

Colditz, G. A., Egan, K. M., & Stampfer, M. J. (1993). Hormone replacement therapy and risk of breast cancer: Results from epidemiologic studies. *American Journal of Obstetrics & Gynecology, 168,* 1473-1480.

Colditz, G. A., Hankinson, S. E., Hunter, D. J., Willett, W. C., Manson, J. E., Stampfer, M. J., Hennekens, C., Rosner, B., & Speizer, F. E. (1995). The use of estrogens and progestins and the risk of breast cancer in postmenopausal women. *New England Journal of Medicine, 332,* 1589-1593.

Collaborative Group on Hormonal Factors in Breast Cancer. (1997). Breast cancer and hormone replacement therapy: Collaborative reanalysis of data from 51 epidemiological studies of 52,807 women with breast cancer and 108,411 women without breast cancer. *Lancet, 350,* 1047-1059.

Colley, C. A., & Lucas, L. M. (1993). Poly-pharmacy: The cure becomes the disease. *Journal of General Internal Medicine, 8*(5), 278-283.

Collier, D. H., & Arend, W. P. (1996). Musculoskeletal diseases. In D. W. Jahnigen & R. W. Schrier (Eds.), *Geriatric medicine* (2nd ed., pp. 558-587). Cambridge, MA: Blackwell.

Collins, T. (1995). Models of health: Pervasive, persuasive and politically charged. *Health Promotion International, 10,* 317-324.

Cominellis, N. (1993). Prevention—The forgotten reform. *Missouri Medicine, 90,* 707-710.

Committee on Diet and Health, Food and Nutrition Board. (1989). *National Research Council: Diet and health: Implications for reducing chronic disease risk.* Washington, DC: National Academy Press.

Council on Scientific Affairs. (1989). Dietary fiber and health. *Journal of the American Medical Association, 262,* 542-546.

Coupland, C., Wood, D., & Cooper, C. (1993). Physical inactivity is an independent risk factor for hip fracture in the elderly. *Journal of Epidemiology and Community Health, 47,* 441-443.

Cuellar, J. (1990). *Aging and health: American Indian/Alaska native* (SGEC Working Paper Series No. 6: Ethnographic Reviews). Stanford, CA: Stanford Geriatric Education Center.

Dalziel, K. L., & Bickers, D. R. (1992). Skin aging. In J. C. Brocklehurst, R. C. Tallis, & H. M. Fillit (Eds.), *Textbook of geriatric medicine and gerontology* (4th ed., pp. 898-926). Edinburgh, Scotland: ChurchHill Living Stone.

D'Angelo, A., & Selhub, J. (1997). Homocysteine and thrombotic disease. *Blood, 90*(1), 1-11.

Dattilo, A. M., & Kris-Etherton, M. (1992). Effects of weight reduction on blood lipids and lopoproteins: A meta-analysis. *American Journal of Clinical Nutrition, 56,* 320-328.

Daviglus, M. L., Stamler, J., Orencia, A. J., Dyer, A. R., Liu, K., Greenland, P., Walsh, M. K., Morris, D., & Shekelle, R. B. (1997). Fish consumption and the 30-year risk of fatal myocardial infarction. *New England Journal of Medicine, 336,* 1046-1053.

DeHoog, S. (1996). The assessment of nutritional status. In L. K. Mahan & S. Escott-Stump (Eds.), *Food, nutrition, and diet therapy* (pp. 361-386). Philadelphia: W. B. Saunders.

Dempster, D. W., & Lindsay, R. (1993). Pathogenesis of osteoporosis. *Lancet, 341,* 797-801.

Dengel, D. R., Hagberg, J. M., Coon, P. J., Drinkwater, D. T., & Goldberg, A. P. (1994). Comparable effects of diet and exercise on body composition and lipoproteins in older men. *Medicine and Science in Sports and Exercise, 26,* 1307-1315.

Despres, J. P., Bouchard, C., Savard, R., Tremblay, A., Marcotte, M., & Theriault, G. (1984). The effect of a 20 week endurance training program on adipose tissue morphology and lipolysis in men and women. *Metabolism, 33,* 235-239.

DiClemente, C. C., & Prochaska, J. O. (1983). Self change and therapy change of smoking behavior: A comparison of processes of change in cessation and maintenance. *Addictive Behaviors, 7,* 133-142.

Dishman, R. K. (1990). Determinants of participation in regular physical activity. In C. Bouchard, R. J. Shephard, T. Stephens, J. R. Sutton, & B. D. McPherson (Eds.), *Exercise, fitness and health* (pp. 214-238). Champaign, IL: Human Kinetics.

Dobbs, A. R., & Rule, B. G. (1989). Adult age: Differences in working memory. *Psychology & Aging, 4,* 500-503.

Dolecek, T. A. (1992). Epidemiological evidence of relationships between dietary polyunsaturated fatty acids and mortality in the multiple risk factor intervention trial. *Proceedings of the Society for Experimental Biology and Medicine, 200,* 177-182.

Downton, J. H., & Andrews, K. (1990). Postural disturbances and psychological symptoms amongst elderly people living at home. *International Journal of Geriatric Psychiatry, 5,* 93-98.

Dracup, K. (1994). Cardiac rehabilitation: The role of social support in recovery and compliance. In S. A. Shumaker & S. M. Czajowski (Eds.), *Social support and cardiovascular disease* (pp. 333-353). New York: Plenum.

Dreosti, I. E. D. (1996). Bioactive ingredients: Antioxidants and polyphenols in tea. *Nutrition Reviews, 54*(11), 51-58.

Dwyer, J. T., Goldin, B. R., Saul, N., Gualtieri, L., Barakat, S., & Adlercreutz, H. (1994). Tofu and soy drinks contain phytoestrogens. *Journal of the American Dietetic Association, 94,* 739-743.

Dzewaltowski, D. A. (1994). Physical activity determinants: A social cognitive approach. *Medicine and Science in Sports and Exercise, 26,* 1395-1399.

Eaker, E. D. (1989). Psychosocial factors in the epidemiology of coronary heart disease in women. *Psychiatric Clinics of North America, 12,* 167-173.

Elder, J. P., Williams, S. J, Drew, J. A., Wright, B. L., & Boulan, T. E. (1995). Longitudinal effects of preventive services on health behaviors among an elderly cohort. *American Journal of Preventive Medicine, 11,* 354-359.

Eley, J. W., Hill, H. A., Chen, V. W., Austin, D. F., Wesley, M. N., Muss, H. B., Greenberg, R. S., Coates, R. J., Correa, P., Redmond, C. K., Hunter, C. P., Herman, A. A., Kurman, R., Blacklow, R., Shapiro, S., & Edwards, B. K. (1994). Racial differences in survival from breast cancer: Results of the National Cancer Institute Black/White Cancer Survival Study. *Journal of the American Medical Association, 272,* 947-954.

Elia, E. A. (1991). Exercise and the elderly. *Clinics in Sports Medicine, 10,* 141-155.

Elward, K., & Larson, E. B. (1992). Benefits of exercise for older adults. *Clinics in Geriatric Medicine, 8,* 35-50.

Eng, E., Salmon, M. E., & Mullan, F. (1992). Community empowerment: The critical base for primary care. *Family and Community Health, 15,* 1-12.

Enstrom, J. E., Kanim, L. E., & Klein, M. A. (1992). Vitamin C intake and mortality among a sample of the United States population. *Epidemiology, 136,* 185.

Esterbauer, H., Dieber-Rotheneder, M., Striegel, M., & Waeg, G. (1991). Role of vitamin E in preventing the oxidation of low density lipoprotein. *American Journal of Clinical Nutrition, 53*(Suppl. 1), 314-321.

Evans, W., & Rosenberg, I. H. (1991). *Biomarkers: The 10 determinants of aging you can control.* New York: Simon & Schuster.

Fain, J. A. (1999). Diabetes. In N. Jairath (Ed.), *Coronary heart disease and risk factor management* (pp. 221-230). Philadelphia: W. B. Saunders.

Farquhar, J. W., Fortmann, S. P., Flora, J. A., Taylor, C. B., & Haskell, W. L. (1990). Effects of community-wide education on cardiovascular disease risk factors. *Journal of the American Medical Association, 264,* 359-365.

Farrell, S. W., Kohl, H. W., & Rogers, T. (1987). The independent effect of ethnicity on cardiovascular fitness. *Human Biology, 59,* 657-666.

Federman, D. G., Concato, J., Caralis, P. V., Hunkele, G. E., & Kirsner, R. S. (1997). Screening for skin cancer in primary care settings. *Archives of Dermatology, 133,* 1423-1425.

Fenstermaker, K. L., Plowman, S. A., & Looney, M. A. (1992). Validation of the Rockport Fitness Walking Test in females 65 years and older. *Research Quarterly for Exercise and Sport, 63,* 322-327.

Ferrini, R., & Barrett-Connor, E. (1996). Caffeine intake and endogenous sex steroid levels in postmenopausal women: The Rancho Bernardo Study. *American Journal of Epidemiology, 144,* 642-644.

Ferrini, R., Edelstein, S., & Barrett-Connor, E. (1994). The association between health beliefs and health behavior change in older adults. *Preventive Medicine, 23*(1), 1-5.

Fiatarone, M. A., & Evans, W. J. (1993). The etiology and reversibility of muscle dysfunction in the aged. *Journal of Gerontology, 348,* 77-83.

Fiatarone, M. A., Marks, E. C., Ryan, N. D., Meredith, C. N., Lipsitz, L. A., & Evans, W. J. (1990). High intensity strength training in nonagenarians: Effects on skeletal muscle. *Journal of the American Medical Association, 263,* 3029-3034.

Fiatarone, M. A., O'Neill, E. F., Ryan, N. D., Clements, K. M., Solares, G. R., Nelson, M. E., Roberts, S. B., Kehayias, J. J., Lipsitz, L. A., & Evans, W. J. (1994). Exercise training and nutritional supplementation for physical frailty in very elderly people. *New England Journal of Medicine, 330,* 1769-1775.

Fillit, H. (1995). Future therapeutic developments of estrogen use. *Journal of Clinical Pharmacology, 35*(Suppl. 9), 25-28.

Fillit, H., & Rowe, J. (1992). The aging kidney. In J. C. Broklehurst, R. C. Tallis, & H. M. Fillit (Eds.), *Textbook of geriatric medicine and gerontology* (4th ed., pp. 612-628). Edinburgh, Scotland: ChurchHill Living Stone.

Fiore, M. C. (1992). Trends in cigarette smoking in the United States: The epidemiology of tobacco use. *Medical Clinics of North America, 76,* 289-303.

Fiore, M. C. (1994). Treatment options for smoking in the '90's. *Journal of Clinical Pharmacology, 34*(3), 195-199.

Fiore, M. C., Jorenby, D. E., & Baker, T. B. (1997). Smoking cessation: Principles and practice based upon the AHCPR guideline. *Annals of Behavioral Medicine, 19*(3), 213-219.

Fiore, M. C., Kenford, S. L., Jorenby, D. E., Wetter, D. W., Smith, S. S., & Baker, T. B. (1994). Two studies of the clinical effectiveness of the nicotine patch with different counseling treatments. *Chest, 105,* 524-533.

Fiore, M. C., Smith, S. S., Jorenby, D. E., & Baker, T. B. (1994). The effectiveness of the nicotine patch for smoking cessation. A meta-analysis. *Journal of the American Medical Association, 271,* 1940-1947.

Flack, J. M., Amaro, H., Jenkins, W., Kunitz, S., Levy, J., Mixon, M., & Yu, E. (1995). Epidemiology of minority health. *Health Psychology, 14,* 592-600.

Fletcher, G. F., Balady, G., Froelicher, V. F., Hartley, L. H., Haskell, W. L., & Pollock, M. L. (1995). Exercise standards: A statement for health care professionals from the American Heart Association. *Circulation, 91,* 580-614.

Flynn, B. C., Rider, M., & Ray, D. W. (1991). Healthy cities: The Indiana model of community development in public health. *Health Education Quarterly, 18,* 331-334.

Folsom, A. R., Burke, G. L., Byers, C. L., Hutchinson, R. G., Heiss, G., Flack, J. M., Jacobs, D. R., Jr., & Caan, B. (1991). Implications of obesity for cardiovascular disease in blacks: The CARDIA and ARIC studies. *American Journal of Clinical Nutrition, 53*(Suppl. 6), 1604-1611.

Folsom, A. R., Wu, K. K., Shahar, E., & Davis, C. E. (1993). Association of hemostatic variables with prevalent cardiovascular disease and asymptomatic carotid artery atherosclerosis—The Atherosclerosis Risk in Communities (ARIC) Study Investigators. *Arteriosclerosis and Thrombosis, 13,* 1829-1836.

Food and Nutrition Board. (1989). *Recommended dietary allowances* (10th ed., National Research Council). Washington, DC: National Academy of Sciences.

Food and Nutrition Board. (1998). *Dietary reference intakes for calcium, phosphorus, magnesium, vitamin D, and fluoride* (Committee on the Scientific Evaluation of Dietary Reference Intakes). Washington, DC: National Academy Press.

Ford, E. S., Merritt, R. K., Heath, G. W., Powell, K. E., Washburn, R. A., Kriska, A., & Haile, G. (1991). Physical activity behaviors in lower and higher socioeconomic status populations. *American Journal of Epidemiology, 133,* 1246-1256.

Fortmann, S. P., Williams, P. T., Hulley, S. B., Haskell, W. L., & Farquhar, J. W. (1981). Effect of health education on dietary behavior: The Stanford Three Community Study. *American Journal of Clinical Nutrition, 34,* 2030-2038.

Fosmire, G. J. (1991). Trace metal requirements. In R. Chernoff (Ed.), *Geriatric nutrition* (pp. 77-100). Gaithersburg, MD: Aspen.

Freudenberg, N., Eng, E., Flay, B., Parcel, G., Rogers, T., & Wallerstein, N. (1995). Strengthening individual and community capacity to prevent disease and promote health: In search of relevant theories and principles. *Health Education Quarterly, 22*(3), 290-306.

Fried, L. P., Ettinger, W. H., Lind, B., Newman, A. B., & Gardin, J. (1994). Physical disability in older adults: A physiological approach. *Journal of Clinical Epidemiology, 47,* 747-760.

Fries, J. F., Bloch, D. A., Harrington, H., Richardson, N., & Beck, R. (1993). Two-year results of a randomized controlled trial of a health promotion program in a retiree population: The Bank of America Study. *American Journal of Medicine, 94,* 455-462.

Fries, J. F., Koop, C. E., Beadle, C. E., Cooper, P. P., England, M. J., Greaves, R. F., Sokolov, J. J., & Wright, D. (1993). Reducing health care costs by reducing the need and demand for health services. *New England Journal of Medicine, 329,* 321-325.

Frishman, W. H., Bryzinski, B. S., Coulson, L. R., DeQuattro, V. L., Vlachakis, N. D., Mroczek, W. J., Dukart, G., Goldberg, J. D., Alemayehu, D., & Koury, K. (1994). A multi factorial trial design to assess combination therapy in hypertension: Treatment with Disoprolol and hydrochloro thiagile. *Archives of Internal Medicine, 154,* 1461-1468.

Frontera, W. R., Hughes, V. A., Lutz, K. J., & Evans, W. J. (1991). A cross-sectional study of muscle strength and mass in 45 to 78 yr-old men and women. *Journal of Applied Physiology, 71,* 644-650.

Frontera, W. R., Meredith, C. N., O'Reilly, K. P., & Evans, W. J. (1990). Strength training determinants of $VO_{2\,max}$ in older men. *Journal of Applied Physiology, 68,* 329-333.

Frontera, W. R., Meredith, C. N., O'Reilly, K. P., Knuttgen, H. G., & Evans, W. J. (1988). Strength conditioning in older men: Skeletal muscle hypertrophy and improved function. *Journal of Applied Physiology, 64,* 1038-1044.

Fujimoto, W. Y., Leonetti, D. L., Kinyoun, J. L., Newell-Morris, L., Shuman, W. P., Stolov, W. C., & Wahl, P. W. (1987). Prevalence of diabetes mellitus and impaired glucose tolerance among second-generation Japanese-American men. *Diabetes, 36,* 721-729.

Fukagawa, N. K., & Young, V. R. (1987). Protein and amino acid metabolism and requirements in older persons. *Clinical Geriatric Medicine, 3,* 329-341.

Furner, S. E., Brody, J., & Jankowski, L. (1997). Epidemiology and aging. In C. K. Cassel, H. J. Cohen, E. B. Larson, D. E. Meier, N. M. Resnick, L. Z. Rubenstein, & L. B. Sorensen (Eds.), *Geriatric medicine* (pp. 37-43). New York: Springer.

Gambacciani, M., Spinetti, A., Cappagli, B., Taponeco, F., Felipetto, R., Parrini, D., Cappelli, N., & Fioretti, P. (1993). Effect of ipriflavone administration on bone mass and metabolism in ovariectomized women. *Journal of Endocrinological Investigation, 16,* 333-337.

Garcia, A. W., & King, A. C. (1991). Predicting long-term adherence to aerobic exercise: A comparison of two models. *Journal of Sport & Exercise Psychology, 13,* 394-410.

Garland, C. F., Friedlander, N. J., Barrett-Connor, E., & Khaw, K. T. (1992). Sex hormones and postmenopausal breast cancer: A prospective study in an adult community. *American Journal of Epidemiology, 135,* 1220-1230.

Gersovitz, M., Motil, K., Munro, H. M., Scrimshaw, N. S., & Young, V. R. (1982). Human protein requirements: Assessment of the adequacy of the current recommended dietary allowance for dietary protein in elderly men and women. *American Journal of Clinical Nutrition, 35*(1), 6-14.

Gersten, J. W. (1991). Effect of exercise on muscle function decline with aging. *Western Journal of Medicine, 154,* 579-582.

Gey, K. F. (1998). Inverse correlation of vitamin E and ischemic heart disease. *International Journal of Vitamin Nutrition Resources, 30,* 224-231.

Gibbs, T. (1988). Health seeking behavior of elderly blacks. In J. Jackson, P. Newton, A. Ostfield, D. Savage, & E. L. Schneider (Eds.), *The Black American elderly: Research on physician and psychosocial health* (pp. 282-291). New York: Spring House.

Gilchrest, B. A., & Yaar, M. (1992). Ageing and photoageing of the skin: Observations at the cellular and molecular level. *British Journal of Dermatology, 127*(Suppl. 41), 25-30.

Goldbaum, R., Hertog, M., Brants, K., van Poppel, G., & van den Brandt, P. (1996). Consumption of black tea and cancer risk: A prospective cohort study. *Journal of the National Cancer Institute, 88*(2), 93-100.

Goldfarb, M. T., Ellis, C. N., & Yoorless, J. J. (1997). Dermatoligic diseases and problems. In C. K. Cassel, H. J. Cohen, E. B. Larson, D. E. Meier, N. M. Resnick, L. Z. Rubenstein, & L. B. Sorensen (Eds.), *Geriatric medicine* (3rd ed., pp. 667-681). New York: Springer.

Goodman, R. M., Wheeler, F. C., & Lee, P. R. (1995). Evaluation of the Heart to Heart project: Lessons from a community-based chronic disease prevention project. *American Journal of Health Promotion, 9,* 443-455.

Gordon, D. J., Probstfield, J. L., Garrison, R. J., Neaton, J. D., Castelli, W. P., Knoke, J. D., Jacobs, D. R., Jr., Bangdiwala, S., & Tyroler, H. A. (1989). High-density lipoprotein cholesterol and cardiovascular disease: Four prospective American studies. *Circulation, 79,* 8-15.

Gordon, N. F., Kohl, H. W., & Blair, S. N. (1993). Life style exercise: A new strategy to promote physical activity for adults. *Journal of Cardiopulmonary Rehabilitation, 13,* 161-163.

Green, L. W., & Kreuter, M. W. (1990). Health promotion as a public health strategy for the 1990s. *Annual Review of Public Health, 11,* 319-334.

Grodstein, F., Stampfer, M., Colditz, G., Willet, W., Manson, J., Joffe, M., Rosner, B., Fuchs, C., Hankinson, S., Hunter, D., Hennekens, C., & Speizer, F. (1997). Postmenopausal hormone therapy and mortality. *New England Journal of Medicine, 336,* 1765-1775.

Grundy, S. M. (1994). Guidelines for cholesterol management: Recommendations of the National Cholesterol Education Program's Adult Treatment Panel II. *Heart Disease & Stroke, 3,* 123-127.

Gur, R. C., Gur, R. E., Obrist, W. D., Skolnick, B. E., & Reivich, M. (1987). Age and regional cerebral blood flow at rest and during cognitive activity. *Archives of General Psychiatry, 44,* 617-621.

Guralnik, J. M., & Kaplan, G. A. (1989). Predictors of healthy aging: Prospective evidence from the Alameda County study. *American Journal of Public Health, 79,* 703-708.

Gurwitz, J. H., & Avorn, J. (1991). The ambiguous relation between aging and adverse drug reactions. *Annals of Internal Medicine, 114,* 956-966.

Haber, D. (1996). Strategies to promote the health of older people: An alternative to readiness stages. *Family and Community Health, 19,* 1-10.

Hagberg, J. M. (1994). Exercise assessment of arthritic and elderly individuals. *Baillière's Clinical Rheumatology, 8*(1), 29-52.

Hagberg, J. M., Graves, J. E., Limacher, M., Woods, D. R., Leggett, S. H., Cononie, C., Gruber, J. J., & Pollock, M. L. (1989). Cardiovascular responses of 70- to 79-yr-old men and women to exercise training. *Journal of Applied Physiology, 66,* 2589-2594.

Ham, R. I. (1992). Indicators of poor nutritional health in older Americans. *American Family Physician, 45*(1), 219-228.

Ham, R. J. (1994). The signs and symptoms of poor nutritional status. *Primary Care, 21,* 33-67.

Hansen, E. F., Andersen, L. T., & Von Eyben, F. E. (1993). Cigarette smoking and age at first acute myocardial infarction, and influence of gender and extent of smoking. *American Journal of Cardiology, 71,* 1439-1442.

Hartshorn, E. A., & Tatro, D. S. (1991). Principles of drug interaction. In D. S. Tatro (Ed.), *Drug interaction facts* (pp. 14-26). Philadelphia: J. B. Lippincott.

Haskell, W. L. (1994). Health consequences of physical activity: Understanding and challenges regarding dose-response. *Medicine and Science in Sports and Exercise, 26,* 649-660.

Haskell, W. L., Leon, A. S., Casperson, C. J., Faselicher, V. F., Hagberg, J. M., Harlan, W., Halloszy, J. D., Regensteiner, J. G., Thompson, P. D., Washburn, R. A., & Wilson, P. W. F. (1992). Cardiovascular benefits and assessment of physical activity and physical fitness in adults. *Medical Science & Sports Exercise, 24*(Suppl. 6), 201-220.

Hathcock, J. N. (1997). Vitamins and minerals: Efficacy and safety. *American Journal of Clinical Nutrition, 66,* 427-437.

Havik, O. E., & Maeland, J. G. (1988). Changes in smoking behavior after a myocardial infarction. *Health Psychology, 7,* 403-420.

Hayes, W. C., Myers, E. R., Robinovitch, S. N., Van Den Kroonenberg, A., Courtney, A. C., & McMahon, T. A. (1996). Etiology and prevention of age-related hip fractures. *Bone, 18*(Suppl. 1), 77-86.

Haynes, S. G., & Feinleib, M. (1980). Women, work and coronary heart disease: Prospective findings from the Framingham heart study. *American Journal of Public Health, 70,* 133-141.

Hebert, P. R., Moser, M., Mayer, J., Glynn, R. J., & Hennekens, C. H. (1993). Recent evidence on drug therapy of mild to moderate hypertension and decreased risk of coronary heart disease. *Archives of Internal Medicine, 153,* 578-581.

Hecht, M., Collier, M. J., & Ribeau, S. (1993). *African American communication: Ethnic identity and cultural interpretations.* Newbury Park, CA: Sage.

Hedegaard, H. B., Davidson, A. J., & Wright, R. A. (1996). Factors associated with screening mammography in low-income women. *American Journal of Preventive Medicine, 12*(1), 51-56.

Helmers, K. F., Krantz, D. S., Howell, R. H., Klein, J., Bairey, C. N., & Rozanski, A. (1993). Hostility and myocardial ischemia in coronary artery disease patients: Evaluation by gender and ischemic index. *Psychosomatic Medicine, 55,* 29-36.

Henningfield, J. E. (1990, January). Understanding nicotine addiction and physical withdrawal process. *Journal of the American Dental Association,* 2S-6S.

Henningfield, J. E., Obarzane, K. E., Benowitz, N. L., Hall, S. M., Klesges, R. C., Leischow, S., Levin, E. D., Perkins, K. A., Spring, B., Stitzer, M., Ward, M. M., Winders, S., Wood, P., Woods, M. N., Isbell, T., & Klem, M. L. (1992). National working conference on smoking and body weight. Task force 2: Methods of assessment, strategies for research. *Health Psychology, 11,* 10-16.

Herings, R. M., Stricker, B. H., de Boer, A., Bakker, A., & Sturmans, F. (1995). Benzodiazepines and the risk of falling leading to femur fractures: Dosage more important than elimination half-life. *Archives of Internal Medicine, 155,* 1801-1807.

Hermanson, B., Omenn, G. S., Kronmal, R. A., & Gersh, B. J. (1988). Beneficial six-year outcome of smoking cessation in older men and women with coronary artery disease. Results from the CASS registry. *New England Journal of Medicine, 319,* 1365-1369.

Hersey, W. C., 3rd, Graves, J. E., Pollock, M. L., Gingerich, R., Shireman, R. B., Heath, G. W., Spierto, F., McCole, S. D., & Hagberg, J. M. (1994). Endurance exercise training improves body composition and plasma insulin response in 70-79 year old men and women. *Metabolism, 43,* 847-854.

Hertog, M. G., Fesdens, E. J., Hollman, P. C., Katan, M. B., & Kromhout, D. (1993). Dietary antioxidant flavonoids and risk of coronary heart disease: The Zutphen elderly study. *Lancet, 342,* 1007-1011.

Hickey, T., Speers, M. A., & Prohaska, T. R. (1997). *Public health and aging.* Baltimore: Johns Hopkins University Press.

Higgins, M. W., Enright, P. L., Kronmal, R. A., Schenker, M. B., Anton-Culver, H., & Lyles, M. (1993). Smoking and lung function in elderly men and women: The cardiovascular health study. *Journal of the American Medical Association, 269,* 2741-2748.

Hill, R. D., Storandt, M., & Malley, M. (1993). The impact of long-term exercise training on psychological function in older adults. *Journal of Gerontology, 48,* 12-17.

Hjalmarson, A., Franzon, M., Westin, A., & Wiklund, O. (1994). Effect of nicotine spray on smoking cessation: A randomized, placebo-controlled, double-blind study. *Archives of Internal Medicine, 154,* 2567-2572.

Ho, S. C., Bacon, W. E., Harris, T., Looker, A., & Magi, S. (1993). Hip fracture rates in Hong Kong and the United States, 1988 through 1989. *American Journal of Public Health, 83,* 694-697.

Hobbs, H. H., Brown, M. S., & Goldstein, J. L. (1992). Molecular genetics of the LDL receptor gene in familial hypercholesterolemia. *Human Mutation, 1,* 445-466.

Hodis, H. N., Mack, W. J., & La Bree, L. (1995). Serial coronary angiographic evidence that antioxidant vitamin intake reduces progression of coronary atherosclerosis. *Journal of the American Medical Association, 273,* 1849-1854.

Holick, M. (1994). McCollum Award Lecture: Vitamin D—New horizions for the 21st century. *American Journal of Clinical Nutrition, 60,* 619.

Hoover, P., Webber, C., Beaumont, L., & Blake, J. (1996). Postmenopausal bone mineral density: Relationship to calcium intake, calcium absorption, residual estrogen, body composition and physical activity. *Canadian Journal of Physiological Pharmacology, 74,* 911-917.

Hopkins, P. N., & Williams, R. R. (1989). Human genetics and coronary heart disease: A public health perspective. *Annual Review of Nutrition, 9,* 303-345.

Hopper, S. V. (1993). The influence of ethnicity on the health of older women. *Clinical Geriatric Medicine, 9*(1), 231-259.

Hornbrook, M. C., Stevens, V. J., Wingfield, D. J., Hollis, J. F., Greenlick, M. R., Ory, M. G., Hubert, H. B., Feinleib, M., McNamara, P. M., & Castelli, W. P. (1994). Preventing falls among community-dwelling older persons: Results from a randomized trial. *Gerontologist, 34,* 16-23.

Horwath, C. C. (1991). Nutrition goals for older adults: A review. *Gerontologist, 31,* 811-821.

Huang, K., Me, I., Wang, Z., Ho, C., Lou, Y., Wang, C., Hard, G., & Conney, A. (1997). Effects of tea, decaffeinated tea, and caffeine on UVB light-induced complete carcinogenesis in SKH-1 mice: Demonstration of caffeine as a biologically important constituent of tea. *Cancer Research, 57,* 2623-2629.

Hubert, H. B., Feinleib, M., McNamara, P. M., & Castelli, W. P. (1983). Obesity as an independent risk factor for cardiovascular disease: A 26-year follow-up of participants in the Framingham Heart Study. *Circulation, 67,* 968-977.

Hughes, J. R. (1995). Combining behavioral therapy and pharmacotherapy for smoking cessation: An update. *NIDA Research Monographs, 150,* 92-109.

Hughes, J. R. (1996). The future of smoking cessation therapy in the United States. *Addiction, 91,* 1797-1802.

Hulley, S. B., & Newman, T. B. (1994). Cholesterol in the elderly: Is it important? *Journal of the American Medical Association, 272,* 1372-1374.

Hunt, S. C., Williams, R. R., & Barlow, G. K. (1986). A comparison of positive family history definitions for defining risk of future disease. *Journal of Chronic Diseases, 39,* 809-821.

Institute of Medicine. (1993). *The future of public health.* Washington, DC: National Academy Press.

Insua, J. T., Sacks, H. S., Lau, T. S., Reitman, D., Pagano, D., & Chalmers, T. C. (1994). Drug treatment of hypertension in the elderly: A meta-analysis. *Annals of Internal Medicine, 121,* 355-362.

Iscoe, I. (1974). Community psychology and the competent community. *American Psychologist, 29,* 607-613.

Ishikawa, T., Suzukawa, M., Ito, T., Yoshida, H., Ayaori, M., Nishiwaki, M., Yoremura, A., Hara, Y., & Nakamura, H. (1997). Effect of tea flavonoid supplementation on the susceptibility of low-density lipoprotein to oxidative modification. *American Journal of Clinical Nutrition, 66,* 261-266.

Jacob, R. A., Wu, M. M., Henning, S. M., & Swendseid, M. E. (1994). Homocysteine increases as folate decreases in plasma of healthy men during short-term dietary folate and methyl group restriction. *Journal of Nutrition, 124,* 1072-1080.

Jandak, J., Steiner, M., & Richardson, P. D. (1989). Alpha-tocopherol, an effective inhibitor of platelet adhesion. *Blood, 73,* 141-149.

Jebb, S. A. (1997). Aetiology of obesity. *British Medical Bulletin, 53,* 264-285.

Jha, P., Flather, M., Lonn, E., Farkouh, M., & Yusuf, S. (1995). The antioxidant vitamins and cardiovascular disease: A critical review of epidemiologic and clinical trial data. *Annals of Internal Medicine, 123,* 860-872.

Johnell, O., Gullberg, B., Kanis, J., Allander, E., Elffors, L., Dequecker, J., Dilsen, G., Gennari, C., Lopes, V., & Lyritis, G. (1995). Risk factors for hip fracture in European women: The MEDOS Study. Mediterranean Osteoporosis Study. *Journal of Bone & Mineral Research, 10,* 1802-1815.

Johnson, B. D., & Dempsey, J. A. (1991). Demand vs. capacity in the aging pulmonary system. *Exercise and Sport Sciences Reviews, 19,* 171-210.

Johnson, K. W., Anderson, N. B., Bastida, E., Kramer, B. J., Williams, D., & Wong, M. (1995). Macrosocial and environmental influences on minority health. *Health Psychology, 14,* 601-612.

Joint National Committee VI. (1997). *The sixth report of the joint national committee on prevention, detection, evaluation and treatment of high blood pressure* (NIH Publication No. 1098-4080, National Institutes of Health; National Heart, Lung and Blood Institute; National High Blood Pressure Education Program). Washington, DC: Author.

Kahn, H. S., Williamson, D. F., & Stevens, J. A. (1991). Race and weight change in U.S. women: The roles of socioeconomic and marital status. *American Journal of Public Health, 81,* 319-323.

Kaiser, F. E., Wilson, M. M. G., & Morley, J. E. (1997). Menopause female sexual function. In C. K. Cassel, H. J. Cohen, E. B. Larson, D. E. Meier, N. M. Resnick, L. Z. Rubenstein, & L. B. Sorensen (Eds.), *Geriatric medicine* (3rd ed., pp. 527-540). New York: Springer.

Kamarck, T. W., & Lichtenstein, E. (1988). Program adherence and coping strategies as predictors of success in a smoking treatment program. *Health Psychology, 7,* 557-574.

Kane, R. A. (1990). Instruments to assess functional status. In C. K. Cassel, D. E. Riesenberg, L. B. Sorensen, & J. R. Walsh (Eds.), *Geriatric medicine* (2nd ed., pp. 169-179). New York: Springer.

Kannel, W. B. (1990). CHD risk factors: A Framingham study update. *Hospital Practice, 25,* 119-130.

Kannel, W. B. (1996). Blood pressure as a cardiovascular risk factor: Prevention and treatment. *Journal of the American Medical Association, 275,* 1571-1576.

Kannel, W. B. (1997). Cardiovascular risk factors in the elderly. *Coronary Artery Disease, 8,* 565-575.

Kannel, W. B., & Higgins, M. (1990). Smoking and hypertension as predictors of cardiovascular risk in population studies. *Journal of Hypertension, 8*(Suppl. 8), 3-8.

Kannel, W. B., Wolf, P. A., Castelli, W. P., & D'Agostino, R. B. (1987). Fibrinogen and risk of cardiovascular disease. The Framingham Study. *Journal of the American Medical Association, 258,* 1183-1186.

Kao, P. C., P'eng, F.-K. (1995). How to reduce the risk factors of osteoporosis in Asia. *Clinical Medical Journal, 55,* 209-213.

Kaplan, G. A. (1997). Behavioral, social and socioenvironmental factors adding years to life and life to years. In T. Hickey, M. Speers, & T. Prohaska (Eds.), *Public health and aging* (pp. 37-52). Baltimore: Johns Hopkins University Press.

Kaplan, G. A., Seeman, T. E., Cohen, R. D., Knudsen, L. P., & Guralnik, J. (1987). Mortality among the elderly in the Alameda County Study: Behavioral and demographic risk factors. *American Journal of Public Health, 77,* 307-312.

Kaplan, G., Strawbridge, W., Camacho, T., & Cohen, R. (1993). Factors associated with change in physical functioning in the elderly: A six-year prospective study. *Journal of Aging and Health, 5,* 140-153.

Kaplan, M. S., & Marks, G. (1990). Adverse effects of acculturation: Psychological distress among Mexican American young adults. *Social Science Medicine, 31,* 1313-1319.

Kappus, H., & Diplock, T. (1992). Tolerance and safety of vitamin E: A toxicological position report. *Free Radical Biology Medicine, 13,* 55.

Katz, S., Ford, A. B., Moskowitz, R. S., Jackson, B. A., & Jaffe, M. W. (1963). Studies of illness in the aged. The index of ADL; A standardized measure of biological and psychosocial function. *Journal of the American Medical Association, 185,* 914-919.

Katz, S. J., & Hofer, T. P. (1994). Socioeconomic disparities in preventive care persist despite universal coverage: Breast and cervical cancer screening in Ontario and the United States. *Journal of the American Medical Association, 272,* 530-534.

Kauffman, Y. (1985). Strength training effect in young and aged women. *Archives of Physical Medicine and Rehabilitation, 65,* 223-226.

Kaufman, D. W., Palmer, J. R., de Mouzon, J., Rosenberg, L., Stolley, P. D., Warshauer, M. E., Zauber, A. G., & Shapiro, S. (1991). Estrogen replacement therapy and the risk of breast cancer: Results from the case-control surveillance study. *American Journal of Epidemiology, 134,* 1375-1385.

Kausler, D. H., Wiley, I. G., & Lieberwitz, K. J. (1992). Adult age differences in short-term memory and subsequent long-term memory for actions. *Psychology & Aging, 7,* 309-316.

Kauwell, G. P., Bailey, L. B., Gregory, J. F., 3rd, Bowling, D. W., & Cousins, R. J. (1995). Zinc status is not adversely affected by folic acid supplementation and zinc intake does not impair folate utilization in human subjects. *Journal of Nutrition, 125*(1), 66-72.

Keller, C. S., & Thomas, K. T. (1995). Measurement of body fat and fat distribution. *Journal of Nursing Measurement, 3*(2), 159-174.

Kendig, H. (1990). Comparative perspectives on housing, ageing, and social structure. In R. H. Binstock & L. K. Georges (Eds.), *Handbook of aging and the social sciences.* San Diego, CA: Academic Press.

Kenford, S. L., Fiore, M. C., Jorenby, D. E., Smith, S. S., Wetter, D., & Baker, T. B. (1994). Predicting smoking cessation: Who will quit with and without the nicotine patch. *Journal of the American Medical Association, 271,* 589-594.

Kennedy, E. T., Ohls, J., Carlson, S., & Fleming, K. (1995). The Healthy Eating Index: Design and applications. *Journal of the American Diet Association, 95,* 1103-1108.

Kerner, J. F., Dusenbury, L., & Mandelblatt, J. S. (1993). Poverty and cultural diversity: Challenges for health promotion among the medically underserved. *Annual Review of Public Health, 14,* 355-377.

King, A. C., Taylor, C. B., Haskell, W. L., & Debusk, R. F. (1988). Strategies for increasing early adherence to and long-term maintenance of home-based exercise training in healthy middle-aged men and women. *American Journal of Cardiology, 61,* 6289-6632.

King, A. C., & Tribble, D. L. (1991). The role of exercise in weight reduction in nonathletes. *Sports Medicine, 11,* 331-349.

Kinosian, B. P., & Eisenberg, J. M. (1988). Cutting into cholesterol: Cost-effective alternatives for treating hypercholesterolemia. *Journal of the American Medical Association, 259,* 2249-2254.

Kitzman, D. W., & Edwards, W. D. (1990). Age-related changes in the anatomy of the normal human heart. *Journal of Gerontological Medical Sciences, 45*(2), 33-39.

Knight, D. C., & Eden, J. (1995). Phytoestrogens—A short review. *Maturitas, 22,* 167-175.

Kohlmeier, L., Weterings, K., Steck, S., & Kok, F. (1997). Tea and cancer prevention: An evaluation of the epidemiologic literature. *Nutrition and Cancer, 27*(1), 1-13.

Koltai, D. C., & Chelune, G. J. (1996). Geriatric neuropsychology. In D. W. Jahnigen & R. W. Schrier (Eds.), *Geriatric medicine* (2nd ed., pp. 41-62). Cambridge, MA: Blackwell.

Koro, T. (1990). Physical training in the aged person. *Japanese Circulation Journal, 54,* 1465-1470.

Kottke, T. E., Brekke, M. L., & Solberg, L. I. (1993). Making "time" for preventive services. *Mayo Clinic Proceedings, 68,* 785-791.

Kris-Etherton, P. M. (1990). *Cardiovascular disease: Nutrition for prevention and treatment.* Chicago, IL: The Association.

Kromhout, D., Feskens, E. J. M., & Bowles, C. H. (1995). The protective effect of a small amount of fish on coronary heart disease mortality in an elderly population. *International Journal of Epidemiology, 24,* 340-345.

Krug, L. M., Haire-Joshu, D., & Heady, S. A. (1991). Exercise habits and exercise relapse in persons with non-insulin-dependent diabetes mellitus. *Diabetes Education, 17*(3), 185-188.

Krumholz, H. M., Seeman, T. E., Merrill, S. S., Mendes de Leon, C. F., Vaccarino, V., Silverman, D. I., Tsukahara, R., Ostfeld, A. M., & Berkman, L. F. (1994). Lack of association between cholesterol and coronary heart disease mortality and morbidity and all-cause mortality in persons older than 70 years. *Journal of the American Medical Association, 272,* 1335-1340.

Kumanyika, S. (1990). Diet and chronic disease issues for minority populations. *Journal of Nutrition Education, 22,* 89-96.

Kumanyika, S. K. (1993). Special issues regarding obesity in minority populations. *Annals of Internal Medicine, 119*(7, Pt. 2), 650-654.

Kumanyika, S. K., & Golden, P. M. (1991). Cross-sectional differences in health status in US racial/ethnic minority groups: Potential influence of temporal changes, disease, and life-style transitions. *Ethnic Diseases, 1,* 50-59.

Kumanyika, S. K., Morssink, C., & Agurs, T. (1992). Models for dietary and weight change in African-American women: Identifying cultural components. *Ethnicity and Disease, 2*(2), 166-175.

Kushi, L. H., Folsom, A. R., Prineas, R. J., Mink, P. I., Wu, Y., & Bostick, R. M. (1996). Dietary antioxidant vitamins and death from coronary heart disease in postmenopausal women. *New England Journal of Medicine, 334,* 1156-1162.

LaCroix, A. Z., Guralnik, J. M., Berkman, L. F., Wallace, R. B., & Satterfield, S. (1993). Maintaining mobility in late life: II. Smoking, alcohol consumption, physical activity, and body mass index. *American Journal of Epidemiology, 137,* 858-869.

LaCroix, A. Z., Lang, J., Scherr, P., Wallace, R. B., Cornoni-Huntley, J., Berkman, L., Curb, J. D., Evans, D., & Hennekens, C. H. (1991). Smoking and mortality among older men and women in three communities. *New England Journal of Medicine, 324,* 1619-1625.

Lapidus, L., Bengtsson, C., Larssons, B., Pennert, K., Rybo, E., & Sjostrom, L. (1984). Distribution of adipose tissue and risk of cardiovascular disease and death: A 12-year follow-up of participants in the population study of women in Gothenberg, Sweden. *British Medical Journal, 289,* 1257-1261.

Lapidus, L., Bengtsson, C., & Lissner, L. (1990). Distribution of adipose tissue in relation to cardiovascular and total mortality as observed during 20 years in a prospective population study of women in Gothenburg, Sweden. *Diabetes Research & Clinical Practice, 10*(Suppl. 1), 185-189.

Lapidus, L., Lindstredt, G., Lundberg, P. A., Bengtsson, C., & Gredmark, T. (1986). Concentrations of sex hormone binding globulin and corticosteroid binding globulin in relation to cardiovascular disease and overall mortality in postmenopausal women. *Clinical Chemistry, 11,* 146-152.

LaRosa, J. C., & Cleeman, J. I. (1992). Cholesterol lowering as a treatment for established coronary heart disease. *Circulation, 8,* 1229-1234.

Larson, E. B., Kukull, W. A., Buchner, D., & Reifler, B. V. (1987). Adverse drug reactions associated with global cognitive impairment in elderly persons. *Annals of Internal Medicine, 107,* 169-173.

Larsson, L. (1982). Physical training effects on muscle morphology in sedentary males at different ages. *Medicine Science Sports & Exercise, 14,* 203-206.

LaVeist, T. A. (1992). The political empowerment and health status of African-Americans: Mapping a new territory. *American Journal of Sociology, 97,* 1080-1095.

Lavie, C. J., Milani, R. V., & Littman, A. B. (1993). Benefits of cardiac rehabilitation and exercise training in secondary coronary prevention in the elderly. *Journal of the American College of Cardiology, 22,* 678-683.

Leiter, L. A., Lukaski, H. C., Kenny, D. J., Barnie, A., Camelon, K., Ferguson, R. S., MacLean, S., Simkins, S., Zinman, B., & Cleary, P. A. (1994). The use of bioelectrical impedance analysis (BIA) to estimate body composition in the Diabetes Control and Complications Trial (DCCT). *International Journal of Obesity & Related Metabolic Disorder, 18,* 829-835.

Leon, A. (1991). Recent advances in the management of hypertension. *Journal of Cardiopulmonary Rehabilitation, 11,* 182-191.

Levine, M., & Perkins, D. V. (1997). *Principles of Community Psychology.* New York: Oxford University Press.

Levy, D., & Kannel, W. B. (1988). Cardiovascular risks: New insights from Framingham. *American Heart Journal, 116,* 2664-2667.

Levy, W. C., Cerqueira, M. D., Abrass, I. B., Schwartz, R. S., & Stratton, J. R. (1993). Endurance exercise training augments diastolic filling at rest and during exercise in healthy young and older men. *Circulation, 88,* 116-226.

Lewis, C. E., Raczynski, J., Heath, G., Levinson, R., Hilyer, J. C., Jr., & Cutter, G. R. (1993). Promoting physical activity in low-income African American communities: The PARR project. *Ethnicity and Disease, 3,* 106-118.

Ley, C. J., Lees, B., & Stevenson, J. C. (1992). Sex- and menopause-associated changes in body-fat distribution. *American Journal of Clinical Nutrition, 55,* 950-954.

Leydon, J. J. (1990). Clinical features of aging skin. *British Journal of Dermatology, 122*(Suppl. 35), 1-3.

Lichtman, R. (1996). Perimenopausal and postmenopausal hormone replacement therapy: Part 2. Hormonal regimens and complementary and alternative therapies. *Journal of Nurse Midwifery, 41,* 195-210.

Lindeman, R. D., & Beck, A. A. (1991). Mineral requirements. In R. Chernoff (Ed.), *Geriatric nutrition* (pp. 53-74). Gaithersburg, MD: Aspen.

Lindheim, S. R., Notelovitz, M., Feldman, E. B., Larsen, S., Kahn, F. Y., & Lobo, R. A. (1994). The independent effects of exercise and estrogen on lipids and lipoproteins in postmenopausal women. *Obstetrics and Gynecology, 83,* 167-172.

Lindsay, R. (1993). Prevention and treatment of osteoporosis. *Lancet, 341,* 801-805.

Lindsay, R., Bush, T. L., Grady, D., Speroff, L., & Lobo, R. A. (1996). Therapeutic controversy: Estrogen replacement in menopause. *Journal of Clinical Endocrinology & Metabolism, 81,* 3829-3838.

Linn, M. W., & Linn, B. S. (1982). The Rapid Disability Rating Scale–2. *Journal of the American Geriatric Society, 30,* 378-382.

Lipid Research Clinics Program. (1984). The Lipid Research Clinics Coronary Primary Prevention Trial results: I. Reduction in incidence of coronary heart disease. *Journal of the American Medical Association, 251,* 351-364.

Lipschitz, D. A. (1995). Approaches to the nutritional support of older patients. *Clinics in Geriatric Medicine, 11,* 715-724.

Liu, W. T., & Yu, E. (1985). Asian/Pacific elderly: Mortality differentials, health status and use of health services. *Journal of Applied Gerontology, 4,* 35-64.

Lloyd, T., Rollings, N., Eggli, D. F., Kieselhorst, K., & Chinchilli, V. (1997). Dietary caffeine intake and bone status of postmenopausal women. *American Journal of Clinical Nutrition, 65,* 1826-1830.

Lober, C. W., & Fenske, N. A. (1990). Photoaging and the skin: Its clinical differentiation and meaning. *Geriatrics, 45,* 36-42.

Lohman, T. G. (1992). *Advances in body composition assessment.* (Current issue of Exercise, Science Service, monograph no. 3). Champaign, IL: Human Kenetics.

Lombard, D. N., Lombard, T. N., & Winett, R. A. (1995). Walking to meet health guidelines: The effect of prompting frequency and prompt structure. *Health Psychology, 14*(2), 164-170.

Lord, S. R., Caplan, G. A., & Ward, J. A. (1993). Balance, reaction time, and muscle strength in exercising and non exercising older women: A pilot study. *Archives of Physical Medicine and Rehabilitation, 74,* 837-839.

Lord, S., & Castell, S. (1994a). Effect of exercise on balance, strength and reaction time in older people. *Australian Journal of Physiotherapy, 40,* 83-88.

Lord, S. R., & Castell, S. (1994b). Physical activity program for older persons: Effect on balance, strength, neuromuscular control, and reaction time. *Archives of Physical Medicine and Rehabilitation, 75,* 648-652.

Losonczy, K. G., Harris, T. B., & Havlik, R. J. (1996). Vitamin E and vitamin C supplement use and risk of all-cause and coronary heart disease mortality in older persons: The Established Populations for Epidemiologic Studies of the Elderly. *American Journal of Clinical Nutrition, 64*(2), 190-206.

Lowenthal, D. T., Kirschner, D. A., Scarpace, N. T., Pollock, M., & Graves, J. (1994). Effects of exercise on age and disease. *Southern Medical Journal, 87*(Suppl. 5), 5-12.

Luepker, R. V., Jacobs, D. R., Gillum, R. F., Folsom, A. R., Prineas, R. J., & Blackburn, H. (1985). Population risk of cardiovascular disease: The Minnesota Heart Survey. *Journal of Chronic Diseases, 38,* 671-682.

Lukaski, H. C. (1987). Methods for the assessment of human body composition: Traditional and new. *American Journal of Clinical Nutrition, 46,* 537-556.

Lunell, E., Molander, L., Leischow, S. J., & Fagerstrom, K. O. (1995). Effect of nicotine vapour inhalation on the relief of tobacco withdrawal symptoms. *European Journal of Clinical Pharmacology, 48,* 235-240.

Lynch, S. M., Gaziano, J. M., & Frei, B. (1996). Ascorbic acid and atherosclerotic cardiovascular disease. *Sub-Cellular Biochemistry, 25,* 331-367.

Lyness, J. M., Bruce, M. L., Koenig, H. G., Parmelee, P. A., Schulz, R., Lawton, M. P., & Reynolds, C. F., 3rd. (1996). Depression and medical illness in late life: Report of a symposium. *Journal of the American Geriatric Society, 44*(2), 198-203.

Magaziner, J., Simonsick, E., Kashner, T., Hebel, J. R., & Kenzora, J. E. (1990). Predictors of functional recovery one year following hospital discharge for hip fracture: A prospective study. *Journal of Gerontology, 45,* M101-M107.

Mahoney, F. L., & Barthel, D. W. (1965). Functional evaluation: The Barthel index. *Maryland State Medical Journal, 14,* 61-65.

Maimen, L. A., & Becker, M. H. (1974). The health belief model: Origins and correlates in psychological theory. In M. H. Becker (Ed.), *The health belief model and personal health behavior* (pp. 9-26). Thorofare, NJ: Slack.

Maki, B. E., Holliday, P. J., & Topper, A. K. (1991). Fear of falling and postural performance in the elderly. *Journal of Gerontology, 46*(4), M123-M131.

Maki, B. E., Holliday, P. J., & Topper, A. K. (1994). Deterioration in postural balance may lead to falls: A prospective study of postural balance and risk of falling in an ambulatory and independent elderly population. *Journal of Gerontology, 49*(2), M72-M84.

Malinow, M. R., Duell, P. B., Hess, D. L., Anderson, P. H., Kruger, W. D., Phillipson, B. E., Gluckman, R. A., Block, P. C., & Upson, B. M. (1998). Reduction of plasma homocyst(e)ine levels by breakfast cereal fortified with folic acid in patients with coronary heart disease. *New England Journal of Medicine, 338,* 1009-1015.

Mandelblatt, J., Traxler, M., Lakin, P., Kanetsky, P., & Kao, R. (1993). Targeting breast and cervical cancer screening to elderly poor black women: Who will participate? The Harlem Study Team. *Preventive Medicine, 22*(1), 20-33.

Mandelblatt, J., Traxler, M., Lakin, P., Kanetsky, P., Thomas, L., Chauhan, P., Matseoane, S., & Ramsey, E. (1993). Breast and cervical cancer screening of poor, elderly, black women: Clinical results and implications. The Harlem Study Team. *American Journal of Preventive Medicine, 9*(3), 133-138.

Manolio, T. A., Furberg, C. D., Shemanski, L., Psaty, B. M., O'Leary, D. H., Tracy, R. P., & Bush, T. L. (1993). Progression of coronary artery disease: Associations of postmenopausal estrogen use with cardiovascular disease and its risk factors in older women. *Circulation, 88*, 2163-2171.

Manolio, T. A., Pearson, T. A., Wenger, N. K., Barrett-Connor, E., Payne, G. H., & Harlan, W. R. (1992). Cholesterol and heart disease in older persons and women. Review of an NHLBI workshop. *Annals of Epidemiology, 2*, 161-176.

Manson, J. E., Colditz, G. A., Stampfer, M. J., Willett, W. C., Rosner, B., Monson, R. R., Speizer, F. E., & Hennekens, C. H. (1990). A prospective study of obesity and risk of coronary heart disease in women. *New England Journal of Medicine, 322*, 882-889.

Marckmann, P., Bladbierg, E.-M., & Jespersen, J. (1997). Dietary fish oil (4g daily) and cardiovascular risk markers in healthy men. *Arteriosclerosis, Thrombosis and Vascular Biology, 17*, 3384-3391.

Marcus, B. H., Rossi, J. S., Selby, V. C., Niaura, R. S., & Abrams, D. B. (1992). The stages and processes of exercise adoption and maintenance in a worksite sample. *Health Psychology, 11*, 386-395.

Marcus, B. H., Selby, V. C., Niaura, R. S., & Rossi, I. S. (1992). Self efficacy and the stages of exercise behavior change. *Research Quarterly for Exercise and Sport, 63*, 60-66.

Markides, K. S., & Miranda, M. R. (Eds.). (1997). *Minorities, aging and health.* Thousand Oaks, CA: Sage.

Markides, K. S., & Vernon, S. W. (1984). Aging, sex-role orientation, and adjustment: A three-generation study of Mexican Americans. *Journal of Gerontology, 39*, 586-591.

Marlatt, G. A., & Gordon, J. R. (1985). *Relapse prevention: Maintenance strategies in the treatment of addictive behaviors.* New York: Guilford.

Marsiglio, A., & Holm, K. (1988). Physical conditioning in the aging adult. *Nurse Practitioner, 13*(9), 33-41.

Mashchak, C. A., Kletzky, O. A., Artal, R., & Mishell, D. R., Jr. (1984). The relation of physiological changes to subjective symptoms in postmenopausal women with and without hot flushes. *Maturitas, 6*, 301-308.

Masoro, E. J. (1993) Dietary restriction and aging. *Journal of the American Geriatrics Society, 41*, 994-999.

Matteson, M. A. (1997). Functional assessment of the elderly. *Nurse Practitioner Forum, 8*(3), 91-98.

McArdle, W. D., Katch, F. I., & Katch, V. L. (1991). *Exercise physiology: Energy, nutrition and human performance* (4th ed.). Baltimore: Williams & Wilkins.

McAuley, E. (1993). Self-efficacy and the maintenance of exercise participation in older adults. *Journal of Behavioral Medicine, 16*(1), 103-113.

McAuley, E., & Jacobson, L. (1991). Self efficacy and exercise participation in sedentary adult females. *American Journal of Health Promotion, 5*(3), 185-191.

McAuley, E., Lox, C., & Duncan, T. E. (1993). Long-term maintenance of exercise, self-efficacy, and physiological change in older adults. *Journal of Gerontology, 48*(4), P218-P224.

McAuley, E., Mihalko, S., & Bane, S. (1997). Exercise and self-esteem in middle aged adults: Multidimensional relationships and physical fitness and self-efficacy influences. *Journal of Behavioral Medicine, 20*(1), 67-83.

McCarron, D. A., Morris, C. D., Young, E., Roullet, C., & Drueke, T. (1991). Dietary calcium and blood pressure: Modifying factors in specific populations. *American Journal of Clinical Nutrition, 54*(Suppl. 1), 215-219.

McCarter, R. J. (1995). Role of caloric restriction in the prolongation of life. *Clinical Geriatric Medicine, 11,* 553-565.

McClaran, S. R., Babcock, M. A., Pegelow, D. F., Reddan, W. G., & Dempsey, J. A. (1995). Longitudinal effects of aging on lung function at rest and exercise in healthy active fit elderly adults. *Journal of Applied Physiology, 78,* 1957-1968.

McCormack, P. (1997). Undernutrition in the elderly population living at home in the community: A review of the literature. *Journal of Advanced Nursing, 26,* 856-863.

McGinnis, J. M., & Ballard-Barbash, R. M. (1991). Obesity in minority populations: Policy implications of research. *American Journal of Clinical Nutrition, 53,* 1512S-1514S.

Meier, D. E. (1997). Osteoporosis and other disorders of skeletal aging. In C. K. Cassel, H. J. Cohen, E. B. Larson, D. E. Meier, N. M. Resnick, L. Z. Rubenstein, & L. B. Sorensen (Eds.), *Geriatric medicine* (3rd ed., pp. 411-432). New York: Springer.

Messina, M. (1994). Soy intake and cancer risk: A review of the in vitro and in vivo data. *Nutrition and Cancer, 21,* 113-131.

Meyer, M. H. (1990). Family status and poverty among older women: The gendered distribution of retirement income in the United States. *Social Problems, 37,* 551-563.

Meyers, A. H., Young, Y., & Langlois, J. A. (1996). Prevention of falls in the elderly. *Bone, 18*(Suppl. 1), 87-101.

Michielutte, R., Dignan, M. B., Sharp, P. C., Boxley, I., & Wells, H. B. (1996). Skin cancer prevention and early detection practices in a sample of nurse women. *Preventive Medicine, 25,* 673-683.

Miksicek, R. J. (1993). Commonly occurring plant flavonoids have estrogenic activity. *Molecular Pharmacology, 44,* 37-43.

Miller, D. L., & Weinstock, M. A. (1994). Nonmelanoma skin cancer in the United States: Incidence. *Journal of the American Academy of Dermatology, 30,* 774-778.

Mills, E. M. (1994). The effect of low-intensity aerobic exercise on muscle strength, flexibility, and balance among sedentary elderly persons. *Nursing Research, 43,* 207-211.

Minkler, M. (1990). Improving health through community organizations. In K. Ganz, F. M. Lewis, & B. K. Rimer (Eds.), *Health behavior and health education: Theory, research and practice* (pp. 257-287). San Francisco: Jossey-Bass.

Minkler, M. (1994). Challenges for health promotion in the 1990's: Social inequities, empowerment, negative consequences, and the common good. *American Journal of Health Promotion, 8,* 404-413.

Minkler, M., & Stone, R. (1985). The feminization of poverty and older women. *Gerontologist, 25,* 351-357.

Moellar, J. F., & Mathiowetz, N. A. (1989). *Prescribed medicines: A summary of use and expenditures for Medicare beneficiaries* (Publication No. PHC 89-3448). Rockville, MD: U.S. Department of Health and Human Services.

Monane, M., Monane, S., & Semla, T. (1997). Optimal medication use in elders: Key to successful aging. *Western Journal of Medicine, 167*(4), 233-237.

Moore, C., & Bracegirdle, H. (1994). The effects of a short-term, low intensity exercise programme on the psychological well being of community-dwelling elderly women. *British Journal of Occupational Therapy, 57,* 213-216.

Moore, J. A., Noiva, R., & Wells, I. C. (1984). Selenium concentrations in plasma of patients with arteriographically defined coronary atherosclerosis. *Clinical Chemistry, 30,* 1171-1173.

Moore, J. M., Oddou, W. E., & Leklem, J. E. (1991). Energy need in childhood and adult-onset obese women before and after a nine-month nutrition education and walking program. *International Journal of Obesity, 15,* 337-344.

Morey, M. C., Cowper, P. A., Feussner, J. R., DiPasquale, R. C., Crowley, G. M., Samsa, G. P., & Sullivan, R. J., Jr. (1991). Two-year trends in physical performance following supervised exercise among community-dwelling older veterans. *Journal of the American Geriatric Society, 39,* 986-992.

Mori, T. A., Beilin, L. J., Burke, V., Morris, J., & Ritchie, J. (1997). Interactions between dietary fat, fish, and fish oils and their effects on platelet function in men at risk of cardiovascular disease. *Arteriosclerosis, Thrombosis and Vascular Biology, 17,* 279-286.

Moritani, T., & deVries, H. A. (1980). Potential for gross muscle hypertrophy in older men. *Journal of Gerontology, 35,* 672-682.

Morris, C. D., & McCarron, D. A. (1987). Dietary calcium intake in hypertension. *Hypertension, 10,* 350-352.

Morris, D. L., Kritchevsky, S. B., & Davis, C. E. (1994). Serum carotenoids and coronary heart disease: The Lipid Research Clinics Coronary Primary Prevention

Trial and Follow-up Study. *Journal of the American Medical Association, 272,* 1439-1441.

Morrison, H. I., Schaubel, D., Desmeules, M., & Wigle, D. T. (1996). Serum folate and risk of fatal coronary heart disease. *Journal of the American Medical Association, 275,* 1893-1896.

Moser, D. K. (1994). Social support and cardiac recovery. *Journal of Cardiovascular Nursing, 9,* 27-36.

Mucignat, C., Castiello, U., Umilta, C., & Tradard, V. (1991). Effect of age on the orientation of attention: Effect of changing the interval between signal and stimulus [Abstract]. *Bollettino-Societa Italiana Biologia Sperimentale, 67,* 521-527.

Muller, J. E., Abela, G. S., Nesto, R. W., & Tofler, G. H. (1994). Triggers, acute risk factors and vulnerable plaques: The lexicon of a new frontier. *Journal of the American College of Cardiology, 23,* 809-813.

Muller-Spahn, F., & Hock, C. (1994). Clinical presentation of depression in the elderly. *Gerontology, 40*(Suppl. 1), 10-14.

Mulrow, C. D., Gerety, M. B., Kanten, D., Cornell, J. E., DeNino, L. A., Chiodo, L., Aguilar, C., O'Neil, M. B., Rosenberg, J., & Solis, R. M. (1994). A randomized trial of physical rehabilitation for very frail nursing home residents. *Journal of the American Medical Association, 271,* 519-524.

Munro, H. N., Suter, P. M., & Russell, R. M. (1987). Nutritional requirements of the elderly. *Annual Review of Nutrition, 7,* 23-39.

Murdaugh, C., & Vanderboom, C. (1997). Individual and community models for promoting wellness. *Journal of Cardiovascular Nursing, 11,* 1-14.

Murkies, A. L., Wilcox, G., & Davis, S. R. (1998). Phytoestrogens. *Journal of Clinical Epidemiology and Metabolism, 83,* 297-303.

Myers, H. F., Kagawa-Singer, M., Kumanyika, S. K., Lex, B. W., & Markides, K. S. (1995). Behavioral risk factors related to chronic diseases in ethnic minorities. *Health Psychology, 14,* 613-621.

Nachtigall, L. E., Nachtigall, R. H., Nachtigall, R. D., & Beckman, E. M. (1979). Estrogen replacement therapy II: A prospective study in the relationship to carcinoma and cardiovascular and metabolic problems. *Obstetrics & Gynecology, 54,* 74-79.

National Center for Health Statistics. (1997). *Health in the United States, 1996.* Hyattsville, MD: Public Health Service.

National Cholesterol Education Program. (1996). *Second report of the expert panel on detection, evaluation, and treatment of high blood cholesterol in adults* (NIH Publication No. 93-3096). Bethesda, MD: National Heart Lung Blood Institute.

National Institutes of Health. (1994). Optimal calcium intake. *NIH Consensus Statement,* 1-31.

National Institutes of Health Consensus Development Conference Statement. (1993). Health implications of obesity. *Annals of Internal Medicine, 103,* 1073-1077.

National Research Council. (1989). *Diet and health: Implications for reducing chronic disease risk.* Washington, DC: National Academy Press.

Nestel, P. J., Pomeroy, S. E., Sasahara, T., Yamashita, T., Dart, A. M., Jennings, G. L., Abbey, K., & Cameron, J. D. (1997). Arterial compliance in obese subjects is improved with dietary plant n-3 fatty acid from flaxseed oil despite increased LDL oxidizability. *Arteriosclerosis, Thrombosis and Vascular Biology, 17,* 1163-1170.

Nestel, P. J., Yamashita, T., Sasahara, T., Pomeroy, S., Dart, A., Komescroft, P., Owen, A., & Abbey, M. (1997). Soy isoflavones improve systemic arterial compliance but not plasma lipids in menopausal and perimenopausal women. *Arteriosclerosis, Thrombosis and Vascular Biology, 17,* 3392-3398.

Neugarten, B. L., & Neugarten, D. (1986). Age in the aging society. *Daedalus, 115*(1), 31-49.

Neugarten, B. L., & Reed, S. C. (1997). Social and psychological characteristics. In C. K. Cassel, H. J. Cohen, E. B. Larson, D. E. Meier, N. M. Resnick, L. Z. Rubenstein, & L. B. Sorensen (Eds.), *Geriatric medicine* (3rd ed., pp. 45-53). New York: Springer.

Newcomb, P. A., Longnecker, M. P., Storer, B. E., Mittendorf, R., Baron, J., Clapp, R. W., Bogdan, G., & Willett, W. C. (1995). Long-term hormone replacement therapy and risk of breast cancer in postmenopausal women. *American Journal of Epidemiology, 142,* 788-795.

Nickens, H. W. (1995). The role of race/ethnicity and social class in minority health status. *Health Services Research, 30*(1, Pt. 2), 151-162.

Nieman, D. C., Henson, D. A., Gusewitch, G., Warren, B. J., Dotson, R. C., Butterworth, D. E., & Nehlsen-Cannarella, S. L. (1993). Physical activity and immune function in elderly women. *Medicine and Science in Sports and Exercise, 25,* 823-831.

Nieman, D. C., Warren, B. J., O'Donnell, K. A., Dotson, R. G., Butterworth, D. E., & Henson, D. A. (1993). Physical activity and serum lipids and lipoproteins in elderly women. *Journal of the American Geriatric Association, 41,* 1339-1344.

Nishina, P. M., Johnson, J. P., Naggert, J. K., & Krauss, R. M. (1992). Linkage of atherogenic lipoprotein phenotype to the low density lipoprotein receptor locus on the short arm of chromosome 19. *Proceedings of the National Academy of the Sciences of the USA, 89,* 708-712.

Nolan, L., & O'Malley, K. (1988). Prescribing for the elderly. Part I: Sensitivity of the elderly to adverse drug reactions. *Journal of the American Geriatric Society, 36,* 142-149.

Nutrition Screening Initiative. (1994). *Incorporating nutrition screening and interventions into medical practice: A monograph for physicians.* Washington, DC: Author.

Nutt, J. G. (1997). Abnormalites of posture and gait. In C. K. Cassel, H. J. Cohen, E. B. Larson, D. E. Meier, N. M. Resnick, L. Z. Rubenstein, & L. B. Sorensen (Eds.), *Geriatric medicine* (3rd ed., pp. 939-948). New York: Springer.

Ockene, J. K. (1987). Physician-delivered interventions for smoking cessation: Strategies for increasing effectiveness. *Preventive Medicine, 16,* 723-737.

Ohkura, T., Isse, K., Akazawa, K., Hamamoto, M., Yaoi, Y., & Hagino, N. (1995). Long-term estrogen replacement therapy in female patients with dementia of the Alzheimer type: 7 case reports. *Dementia, 6*(2), 99-107.

Ohlson, L. O., Larsson, B., Svardsudd, K., Welin, L., Eriksson, H., Wilhelmsen, L., Bjorntorp, P., & Tibblin, G. (1985). The influence of body fat distribution on the incidence of diabetes mellitus: 13.5 years of follow-up of the participants in the study of men born in 1913. *Diabetes, 34,* 1055-1058.

Omenn, G. S., Beresford, S. A., Buchner, D. M., LaCroix, A., Martin, M., Patrick, D. L., Wallace, J. T., Wagner, E. H. (1997). Evidence of modifiable risk factors in older adults as a basis for health promotion and disease prevention programs. In T. Hickey, M. A. Speers, & T. R. Prohaska, (Eds.), *Public health and aging.* Baltimore: The Johns Hopkins University Press.

Omenn, G. S., Goodman, G. E., Thornquist, M. D., Balmes, J., Cullen, M. R., Glass, A., Keogh, J. P., Meyskens, F. L., Jr., Valanis, B., Williams, J. H., Jr., Barnhart, S., Cherniack, M. G., Brodkin, C. A., & Hammar, S. (1996). Risk factors for lung cancer and for intervention effects in CARET, the Beta-Carotene and Retinol Efficacy Trial. *Journal of the National Cancer Institute, 88,* 1550-1559.

Opie, L. H. (1997). New developments in cardiovascular drugs: Vitamin E and antioxidants—An informal and personal viewpoint. *Cardiovascular Drugs & Therapy, 11,* 719-721.

Opper, F. H., & Burakoff, R. (1994). Nutritional support of the elderly patient in an intensive care unit. *Clinics in Geriatric Medicine, 10*(1), 31-49.

Orleans, C. T., Resch, N., Noll, E., Keintz, M. K., Rimer, B. K., Brown, T. V., & Snedden, T. M. (1994). Use of transdermal nicotine patch in a state-level prescription plan for the elderly: A first look at "real world" patch users. *Journal of the American Medical Association, 271,* 601-607.

Orth-Gomer, K., Rosengren, A., & Wilhelmsen, L. (1993). Lack of social support and incidence of coronary heart disease in middle-aged Swedish men. *Psychosomatic Medicine, 55,* 37-43.

Orwoll, E. S., Ferar, J., Oviatt, S. K., McClung, M. R., & Huntington, K. (1989). The relationship of swimming exercise to bone mass in men and women. *Archives of Internal Medicine, 149,* 2197-2200.

Owen, N., Bauman, A., Booth, M., Oldenburg, B., & Magnus, P. (1995). Social mass-media campaigns to promote physical activity: Reinforcing or redundant? *American Journal of Public Health, 85,* 244-248.

Owens, J. F., Matthews, K. A., Wing, R. R., & Kuller, L. H. (1990). Physical activity and cardiovascular risk: A cross-sectional study of middle-aged premenopausal women. *Preventive Medicine, 19,* 147-157.

Paffenbarger, R. S., Jr., Hyde, R. T., Wing, A. L., & Hsieh, C. C. (1986). Physical activity, all-cause mortality, and longevity of college alumni. *New England Journal of Medicine, 314,* 605-613.

Paffenbarger, R. S., Jr., Hyde, R. T., Wing, A. L., Lee, I. M., Jung, D. L., & Kampert, J. B. (1993). The association of changes in physical-activity level and other lifestyle characteristics with mortality among men. *New England Journal of Medicine, 328,* 538-545.

Parker, S. L., Tong, T., Bolden, S., & Wingo, P. A. (1996). Cancer statistics, 1996. *California Cancer Journal Clinics, 65,* 5-27.

Pate, R. R., Pratt, M., Blair, S. N., Haskell, W. L., Macera, C. A., Bouchard, C., Buchner, D., Ettinger, W., Heath, G. W., King, A. C., Kriska, A., Leon, A. S., Marcus, B. H., Morris, J., Paffenbarger, R. S., Jr., Patrick, K., Pollock, M. L., Rippe, J. M., Sallis, J., & Wilmore, J. H. (1995). Physical activity and public health. A recommendation from the Centers for Disease Control and Prevention and the American College of Sports Medicine. *Journal of the American Medical Association, 273,* 402-407.

Pearlman, D. N., Rakowski, W., Ehrich, B., & Clark, M. A. (1996). Breast cancer screening practices among black, Hispanic, and white women: Reassessing differences. *American Journal of Preventive Medicine, 12,* 327-337.

Pekkanen, J., Nissinen, A., Vartiainen, E., Salonen, J. T., Punsar, S., Karvonen, M. J. (1994). Changes in serum cholesterol level and mortality: A 30-year follow-up. The Finnish cohorts of the seven countries study. *American Journal of Epidemiology, 139*(2), 155-165.

PEPI Writing Group. (1995). Effects of estrogen or estrogen/progestin regimens on heart disease risk factors in postmenopausal women. The Postmenopausal Estrogen/Progestin Interventions (PEPI) Trial. *Journal of the American Medical Association, 273,* 199-208.

Persson, I., Yuen, J., Bergkvist, L., Adami, H. O., Hoover, R., & Schairer, C. (1992). Combined oestrogen-progestogen replacement and breast cancer risk. *Lancet, 340,* 1044.

Pinholt, E. M., Kroenke, K., Hanley, J. F., Kussman, M. J., Twyman, P. L., & Carpenter, J. L. (1987). Functional assessment of the elderly: A comparison of standard instruments with clinical judgment. *Archives of Internal Medicine, 147,* 484-488.

Pi-Sunyer, F. X. (1993). Short-term medical benefits and adverse effects of weight loss. *Annals of Internal Medicine, 119,* 722-726.

Pitkin, R. M. (1998). What the new dietary recommendations mean for your patients: Spotlight on B vitamins and choline. *Consultant.*

Pollock, M. L., & Jackson, A. S. (1984). Research progress in validation of clinical methods of assessing body composition. *Medicine and Science in Sports and Exercise, 16,* 606-615.

Posner, J. D., Gorman, K. M., Gitlin, L. N., Sands, L. P., Kleban, M., Windsor, L., & Shaw, C. (1990). Effects of exercise training in the elderly on the occurrence and time to onset of cardiovascular diagnoses. *Journal of the American Geriatric Society, 38,* 205-210.

Pratley, R., Nicklas, B., Rubin, M., Miller, J., Smith, A., Smith, M., Hurley, B., & Goldberg, A. (1994). Strength training increases resting metabolic rate and norepinephrine levels in healthy 50- to 65-yr-old men. *Journal of Applied Physiology, 76*(1), 133-137.

Price, K. R., & Fenwick, G. R. (1985). Naturally occurring oestrogens in foods a review. *Food Additives & Contamination, 2,* 73-106.

Prochaska, J. O., & DiClemente, C. C. (1984). Self change processes, self efficacy and decisional balance across five stages of smoking cessation. *Program of Clinical & Biological Research, 156,* 131-140.

Puska, P., Nissinen, A., Tuomilehto, J., Saloven, J. T., & Koskela, K. (1985). The community-based strategy to prevent coronary heart disease: Conclusions from the ten years of the North Karelia project. *Annual Review of Public Health, 6,* 147-193.

Pyykko, I., Jantti, P., & Aalto, H. (1990). Postural control in elderly subjects. *Age and Aging, 19,* 215-221.

Racette, S. B., Schoeller, D. A., Kushner, R. F., Neil, K. M., & Herling-Iaffaldano, K. (1995). Effects of aerobic exercise and dietary carbohydrate on energy expenditure and body composition during weight reduction in obese women. *American Journal of Clinical Nutrition, 61,* 486-494.

Ray, W. A., Griffin, M. R., & Shorr, R. I. (1990). Adverse drug reaction and the elderly. *Health Affairs, 9,* 114-122.

Reaven, G. M. (1993). Role of insulin resistance in human disease (Syndrome X): An expanded definition. *Annual Review of Medicine, 44,* 121-131.

Reaven, G. M. (1995). Pathophysiology of insulin resistance in human disease. *Physiology Review, 75,* 473-476.

Reaven, P. D., Barrett-Connor, E., & Edelstein, S. (1991). Relation between leisure-time physical activity and blood pressure in older women. *Circulation, 83,* 559-565.

Redfoot, D., & Gaberlavage, G. (1991). Housing for older Americans: Sustaining the dream. *Generations, 15,* 35-38.

Renaud, S., & de Lorgeril, M. (1992). Wine, alcohol, platelets, and the French paradox for coronary disease. *Lancet, 339,* 1523-1526.

Resnick, N. M. (1995). Urinary incontinence. *Lancet, 346,* 94-99.

Resnick, N. M., Elbadaw, A., & Yalla, S. V. (1995). Age and the lower urinary tract: What is normal? *Neurological Urodynamics, 14,* 577-579.

Resnick, N. M., & Ouslander, I. G. (Eds.). (1990). National Institute of Health Census development conference on urinary incontinence. *Journal of the American Geriatric Society, 38,* 263-386.

Reuben, D. B., & Siu, A. L. (1990). An objective measure of physical function of elderly outpatients: The Physical Performance Test. *Journal of the American Geriatric Society, 38,* 1105-1112.

Rho, J. P., & Wong, F. S. (1998). Principles of prescribing medications. In T. Yoshikawa, E. Cobbs, & K. Brummel-Smith (Eds.), *Practical ambulatory geriatrics* (2nd ed., pp. 19-25). St. Louis, MO: C. V. Mosby.

Riegel, B. (1989). Social support and psychological adjustment to chronic coronary heart disease: Operationalization of Johnson's behavioral system model. *Advances in Nursing Science, 11,* 74-84.

Ripsin, C. M., Keenan, J. M., Jacobs, D. R., Jr., Elmer, P. J., Welch, R. R., Van Horn, L., Liu, K., Turnball, W. H., Thye, F. W., Kestin, M., Hegsted, M., Davidson, D. M., Davidson, M. H., Dugan, L. D., Demark-Wahnefried, W., & Beling, S. (1992). Oat products and lipid lowering: A meta-analysis. *Journal of the American Medical Association, 267,* 3317-3325.

Roach, M., 3rd, Cirrincione, C., Budman, D., Hayes, D., Berry, D., Younger, J., Hart, R., & Henderson, I. C. (1997). Race and survival from breast cancer: Based on Cancer and Leukemia Group B trial 8541. *Cancer Journal From Scientific American, 3*(2), 107-112.

Robbins, K. (1991, Spring). Heart, body and soul: The gospel of good health. *Hopkins Medical News,* 2-6.

Robinson, B. E. (1998). Depression. *Archives of the American Academy of Orthopaedic Surgeons, 2,* 33-37.

Rogers, E. M. (1995). *Diffusion of innovations* (3rd ed.). New York: Free Press.

Rogers, H. B., Schroeder, T., Secher, N. H., & Mitchell, J. H. (1990). Cerebral blood flow during static exercise in humans. *Journal of Applied Physiology, 68,* 2358-2361.

Rogers, M. A., & Evans, W. J. (1993). Changes in skeletal muscle with aging: Effects of exercise training. *Exercise, Sports and Science Review, 21,* 65-102.

Roos, M. R., Rice, C. L., & Vandervoort, A. A. (1997). Age-related changes in motor unit function. *Muscle Nerve, 20,* 679-690.

Rosenberg, I. H., & Miller, J. W. (1992). Nutrition in the elderly: Symposium on nutrition and aging. *Nutrition Review, 50,* 349.

Rosenstock, I. M. (1974). The health belief model and preventive health behavior. *Health Education Monograph, 2,* 354-383.

Rowe, J. W., & Lipsitz, L. A. (1988). Altered blood pressure. In J. W. Rowe & R. W. Besdine (Eds.), *Geriatric medicine* (2nd ed., pp. 193-207). Boston: Little, Brown.

Rubenstein, L. Z. (1998). Falls. In T. Yoshikawa, E. Cobbs, & K. Brummel-Smith (Eds.), *Practical ambulatory geriatrics* (2nd ed., pp. 262-269). St. Louis, MO: C. V. Mosby.

Rubenstein, L., Robbin, S. A., Josephson, K., Trueblood, P., Wallis, R. A., & Loy, S. (1994). Effects of an exercise intervention on fall-prone elderly men. *Journal of the American Geriatrics Society, 41*(Suppl.), A5.

Rubenstein, L. Z., Wieland, G. D., & Bernabei, R. (1995). *Geriatric assessment technology: The state of the art.* Milan, Italy: Kurtis.

Rudman, D., & Cohan, M. E. (1991). Polyunsaturated fatty acids and the health of the elderly. *World Review of Nutrition & Diet, 66,* 143-160.

Sallis, J. F., & Hovell, M. F. (1990). Determinants of exercise behavior. *Exercise in Sports and Science Review, 18,* 307-330.

Sallis, J. F., Patterson, T. L., Buono, M. J., Atkins, C. J., & Nader, P. R. (1988). Aggregation of physical activity habits in Mexican-American and Anglo families. *Journal of Behavioral Medicine, 11*(1), 31-41.

Salonen, J. T., Alfthan, G., Huttunen, J. K., Pikkarainen, J., & Puska, P. (1982). Association between cardiovascular death and myocardial infarction and serum selenium in a matched-pair longitudinal study. *Lancet, 2,* 175-179.

Salthouse, T. A. (1991). Age and experience effects on the interpretation of orthographic drawings of three-dimensional objects. *Psychology & Aging, 6,* 426-433.

Samsioe, G. (1997). Osteoporosis—An update. *Acta Obstetrics & Gynecolology of Scandinavia, 76*(3), 189-199.

Schaberg-Lorei, G., Ballard, J. E., McKeown, B. C., & Zinkgraf, S. A. (1990). Body composition alterations consequent to an exercise program for pre and post menopausal women. *Journal of Sports Medicine and Physical Fitness, 30,* 426-433.

Scharbo-Dehaan, M. (1996). Hormone replacement therapy. *Nurse Practitioner, 21*(12, Pt. 2), 1-13.

Schmidt, R., Fazekas, F., Reinhart, B., Kapeller, P., Fazekas, G., Offenbacher, H., Eber, B., Schumacher, M., & Freidl, W. (1996). Estrogen replacement therapy in older women: A neuropsychological and brain MRI study. *Journal of the American Geriatrics Society, 44,* 1307-1313.

Schoenborn, C. A., & Marano, M. (1988). Current estimates from the National Health Interview Survey. *Vital Health Statistics, 10*(166), 1-233.

Schoenfeld, D. E., Malmrose, L. C., Blazer, D. G., Gold, D. T., & Seeman, T. E. (1994). Self-rated health and mortality in the high-functioning elderly—A closer look at healthy individuals: MacArthur field study of successful aging. *Journal of Gerontology, 49,* M109-M115.

Schwartz, J., Freeman, R., & Frishman, W. (1995). Clinical pharmacology of estrogens: Cardiovascular actions and cardioprotective benefits of replacement therapy in postmenopausal women. *Journal of Clinical Pharmacology, 35,* 314-329.

Seeman, T., Berkman, L., Kohout, F., Lacroix, A., Glynn, R., & Blazer, D. (1993). Intercommunity variations in the association between social ties and mortality in the elderly: A comparative analysis of three communities. *Annals of Epidemiology, 3,* 325-335.

Seeman, T. E., Kaplan, G. A., Knudsen, L., Cohen, R., & Guralnik, J. (1987). Social network ties and mortality among the elderly in the Alameda County Study. *American Journal of Epidemiology, 126,* 714-723.

Seeman, T. E., & Syme, S. L. (1987). Social networks and coronary artery disease: A comparison of the structure and function of social relations as predictors of disease. *Psychosomatic Medicine, 49,* 341-354.

Selhub, J., Jacques, P. F., Wilson, P. W., Rush, D., & Rosenberg, I. H. (1993). Vitamin status and intake as primary determinants of homocysteinemia in an elderly population. *Journal of the American Medical Association, 270,* 2693-2698.

Sempos, C. T. (1993). The Expert Panel on detection, evaluation and treatment of high blood cholesterol in adults. *Journal of the American Medical Association, 269,* 3009-3014.

Shangold, M. M.(1990). Exercise in the menopausal woman. *Obstetrics and Gynecology, 75*(Suppl. 4), 53-58.

Shapiro, E. D., Berg, A., Austrian, R., Schroeder, D., Parcells, V., Margolis, A., Adair, R. K., & Clemens, J. D. (1991). The protective efficacy of polyvalent pneumoccal polysaccharide vaccine. *New England Journal of Medicine, 325,* 1453-1460.

Sharma, R. D. (1979). Isoflavones and hypercholesterol in rats. *Lipids, 14,* 535-540.

SHEP Cooperative Research Group. (1991). Prevention of stroke by antihypertensive drug treatment in elder persons with isolated systolic hypertension: Final results of the systolic hypertension in the elderly program (SHEP). *Journal of the American Medical Association, 265,* 3255-3264.

Shephard, R. J. (1997). *Aging, physical activity and health.* Champaign, IL: Human Kenetics.

Sherman, S. E., D'Agostino, R. B., Cobb, J. L., & Kannel, W. B. (1994). Does exercise reduce mortality rates in the elderly? Experience from the Framingham Heart Study. *American Heart Journal, 128,* 965-972.

Sherwin, B. B., & Gelf, M. M. (1989). A prospective one-year study of estrogen and progestin in postmenopausal women: Effects on clinical symptoms and lipoprotein lipids. *Obstetrics & Gynecology, 73*(5, Pt. 1), 759-766.

Shimokata, H., Tobin, J. D., Muller, D. C., Elahi, D., Coon, P. J., & Andres, R. (1989). Studies in the distribution of body fat: I. Effects of age, sex, and obesity. *Journal of Gerontology, 44*(2), M66-M73.

Silagy, C., Mant, D., Fowler, G., & Lodge, M. (1994). Meta-analysis on efficacy of nicotine requirement therapies in smoking cessation. *Lancet, 343,* 139-142.

Silver, A. J., & Morley, J. E. (1993). Role of the opioid system in the hypodipsia associated with aging. *Journal of the American Geriatric Society, 40,* 556-560.

Simonsick, E. M., Lafferty, M. E., Phillips, C. L., Mendes de Leon, C. F., Kasl, S. V., Seeman, T. E., Fillenbaum, G., Hebert, P., & Lemke, J. H. (1993). Risk due to inactivity in physically capable older adults. *American Journal of Public Health, 83,* 1443-1450.

Singleton, J. W. (1990). Management of constipation and diarrhea. In R. N. Schrier (Ed.), *Geriatric medicine* (pp. 434-439). Philadelphia: W. B. Saunders.

Sirtori, C. R., Agradi, E., Conto, F., Mantero, O., & Gatti, E. (1977). Soybean-protein diet in the treatment of type-II hyperlipogroteinemia. *Lancet, 1,* 275-277.

Siscovick, D. S., King, I., Weinmann, S., Lemaitre. R., Raghunathan, T. E., Psaty, B., Cobb, L., Retzlaff, B., & Knopp, R. (1995). Dietary intake and cell membrane levels of long-chain n-3 polyunsaturated fatty acids and the risk of primary cardiac arrest. *Journal of the American Medical Association, 274,* 1363-1367.

Slemenda, C. W., Miller, J. Z., Hui, S. L., Reister, T. K., & Johnston, C. C., Jr. (1991). Role of physical activity in the development of skeletal mass in children. *Journal of Bone Mineral Research, 6,* 1227-1233.

Smith, E. L., Reddan, W., & Smith, P. E. (1981). Physical activity and calcium modalities for bone mineral increase in aged women. *Medicine and Science in Sports and Exercise, 13,* 60-64.

Smith, G. E., Malec, J. F., & Ivnik, R. J. (1992). Validity of the construct of nonverbal memory: A factor analytic study in a normal elderly sample. *Journal of Clinical and Experimental Neuropsychology, 14,* 211-221.

Sonstroem, R. J., & Morgan, W. P. (1989). Exercise and self-esteem: Rationale and model. *Medicine and Science in Sports and Exercise, 21,* 329-337.

Sorock, G. S., Bush, T. L., Golden, A. L., Fried, L. P., Breuer, B., & Hale, W. E. (1988). Physical activity and fracture risk in a free-living elderly cohort. *Journal of Gerontology, Medicine and Science, 43,* 134-139.

Soules, M. R., & Bremner, W. J. (1982). The menopause and climacteric: Endocrinologic basis and associated symptomatology. *Journal of the American Geriatric Society, 30,* 547-561.

Speroff, L. (1996). Postmenopausal hormone therapy and breast cancer. *Obstetrics and Gynecology, 87*(Suppl. 2), 44-54.

Srebnik, D. S. (1991). Principles of community psychology. *The Community Psychologist, 24,* 8.

Stahl, W., & Sies, H. (1997). Antioxidant defense: Vitamins E and C and carotenoids. *Diabetes, 46*(Suppl. 2), 14-18.

Stampfer, M. J., & Colditz, G. A. (1991). Estrogen replacement therapy and coronary heart disease: A quantitative assessment of the epidemiologic evidence. *Preventive Medicine, 20*(1), 47-63.

Stampfer, M. J., Hennekens, C. H., Manson, J. E., Colditz, G. A., Rosner, B., & Willett, W. C. (1993). Vitamin E consumption and the risk of coronary disease in women. *New England Journal of Medicine, 328,* 1444-1449.

Stampfer, M. J., Malinow, M. R., Willett, W. C., Newcomer, L. M., Upson, B., Ullmann, D., Tishler, P. V., & Hennekens, C. H. (1992). A prospective study of plasma homocysteine and risk of myocardial infarction. *Journal of the American Medical Association, 268,* 877-881.

Stanford, J. L., Weiss, N. S., Voigt, L. F., Daling, J. R., Habel, L. A., & Rossing, M. A. (1995). Combined estrogen and progestin hormone replacement therapy in relation to risk of breast cancer in middle-aged women. *Journal of the American Medical Association, 274,* 137-142.

Staudinger, U. M., Marsiske, M., & Baltes, P. B. (1993). Resilience and levels of reserve capacity in later adulthood: Perspectives from life-span theory. *Development and Psychopathology, 5,* 541-566.

Stavig, G. R., Igra, A., & Leonard, A. R. (1988). Hypertension and related health issues among Asians and Pacific Islanders in California. *Public Health Report, 103*(1), 28-37.

Stefanick, M. L., Legault, C., Tracy, R. P., Howard, G., Kessler, C. M., Lucas, D. L., & Bush, T. L. (1995). Distribution and correlates of plasma fibrinogen in middle-aged women: Initial findings of the postmenopausal estrogen/progestin interventions (PEPI) study. *Arteriosclerosis, Thrombosis and Vascular Biology, 15,* 2085-2093.

Steinbach, U. (1992). Social networks, institutionalization, and mortality among elderly people in the United States. *Journal of Gerontology, 47,* S183-S190.

Steinberg, K. K., Thacker, S. B., Smith, S. J., Stroup, D. F., Zack, M. M., Flanders, W. D., & Berkelman, R. L. (1991). A meta-analysis of the effect of estrogen replacement therapy on the risk of breast cancer. *Journal of the American Medical Association, 265,* 1985-1990.

Steiner, M. (1993). Vitamin E and the risk of coronary disease. *New England Journal of Medicine, 329,* 1424-1425.

Steinhaus, L. A., Dustman, R. E., Ruhling, R. O., Emmerson, R. Y., Johnson, S. C., Shearer, D. E., Latin, R. W., Shigeoka, J. W., & Bonekat, W. H. (1990). Aerobic capacity of older adults: A training study. *Journal of Sports Medicine and Physical Fitness, 30*(2), 163-172.

Stelmach, G. E., Populin, L., & Muller, F. (1990). Postural muscle onset and voluntary movement in the elderly. *Neuroscience Letters, 117,* 188-193.

Stephens, N. G., Parsons, A., & Schofield, P. M. (1996). Randomized controlled trial of vitamin E in patients with coronary disease. Cambridge Heart Antioxidant Study (CHAOS). *Lancet, 347,* 781-786.

Stevenson, J. S., & Topp, R. (1990). Effects of moderate and low intensity long-term exercise by older adults. *Research in Nursing Health, 13,* 209-218.

Stewart, D. E., & Boydell, K. M. (1993). Psychologic distress during menopause: Associations across the reproductive life cycle. *International Journal of Psychiatry Medicine, 23,* 157-162.

Stokols, D. (1992). Establishing and maintaining health environments: Toward a social ecology of health promotion. *American Psychologist, 47,* 6-22.

Stokols, D. (1996). Translating social ecological theory into guidelines for community health promotion. *American Journal of Health Promotion, 10,* 282-298.

Stollerman, G. H., (1997). Infectious disease. In C. K. Cassel, H. J. Cohen, E. B. Larson, D. E. Meier, N. M. Resnick, L. Z. Rubenstein, & L. B. Sorensen (Eds.), *Geriatric medicine* (3rd ed., pp. 599-656). New York: Springer.

Sugarman, J. R., Warren, C. W., Oge, L., & Helgerson, S. D. (1992). Using the Behavioral Risk Factor Surveillance System to monitor year 2000 objectives among American Indians. *Public Health Report, 107,* 449-456.

Sugisawa, H., Liang, J., & Liu, X. (1994). Social networks, social support, and mortality among older people in Japan. *Journal of Gerontology, 49*(Suppl. 1), 3-13.

Sullivan, D. H., Walls, R. C., & Lipschitz, D. A. (1991). Protein-energy undernutrition and the risk of mortality within 1 year of hospital discharge in a select population of geriatric rehabilitation patients. *American Journal of Clinical Nutrition, 53,* 599-605.

Sullivan, J. M., Vander Zwaag, R., Hughes, J. P., Maddock, V., Kroetz, F. W., Ramanathan, K. B., & Mirvis, D. M. (1990). Estrogen replacement and coronary artery disease: Effect on survival in postmenopausal women. *Archives of Internal Medicine, 150,* 2557-2562.

Suter, P. M. (1991). Vitamin requirements. In R. Chernoff (Ed.), *Geriatric nutrition* (pp. 25-42). Gaithersburg, MD, Aspen.

Svendsen, O. L., Hassager, C., & Christiansen, C. (1994). Six month's follow-up on exercise added to a short-term diet in overweight postmenopausal women— Effects on body composition, resting metabolic rate, cardiovascular risk factors and bone. *International Journal of Obesity, 18,* 692-696.

Szklo, M., Cerhan, J., Diez-Roux, A. V., Chambless, L., Cooper, L., Folsom, A. R., Fried, L. P., Knopman, D., & Nieto, F. J. (1996). Estrogen replacement therapy and cognitive functioning in the Atherosclerosis Risk in Communities (ARIC) Study. *American Journal of Epidemiology, 144,* 1048-1057.

Taaffe, D. R., Pruitt, L., Reim, J., Butterfield, G., & Marcus, R. (1993). Effect of sustained resistance training on basal metabolic rate in older women. *Journal of the American Geriatric Society, 43,* 465-471.

Tate, C. A., Hyek, M. F., & Taffet, G. E. (1994). Mechanisms for the responses of cardiac muscle to physical activity in old age. *Medicine and Science in Sports and Exercise, 26,* 561-567.

Taylor, M. (1997). Alternatives to conventional hormone replacement therapy. *Comprehensive Therapy, 23,* 514-532.

Thompson, R. F., Crist, D. M., Marsh, M., & Rosenthal, M. (1988). Effects of physical exercise for elderly patients with physical impairments. *Journal of the American Geriatric Society, 36,* 130-135.

Tinetti, M. E., Baker, D. I., McAvay, G., Claus, E. B., Garrett, P., Gottschalk, M., Koch, M. L., Trainor, K., & Horwitz, R. I. (1994). A multifactorial intervention to reduce the risk of falling among elderly people living in the community. *New England Journal of Medicine, 331,* 821-827.

Tinetti, M. E., Speechley, M., & Ginter, S. F. (1988). Risk factors for falls among elderly persons living in the community. *New England Journal of Medicine, 319,* 1701-1707.

Tonnesen, P., Norregaard, J., Simonson, K., & Sawe, U. (1992). A double-blind trail of nicotine patches in smoking cessation. *Ugeskrift for haeger, 154*(5), 251-254.

Tremblay, A., Despres, J. P., Maheux, J., Pouliot, M. C., Nadeau, A., Moorjani, S., Lupien, P. J., & Bouchard, C. (1991). Normalization of the metabolic profile in obese women by exercise and a low fat diet. *Medicine and Science in Sports and Exercise, 23,* 1326-1331.

Tuck, M. L., Sowers, J., & Dornfeld, L. (1981). The effect of weight reduction on blood pressure, plasma renin activity, and plasma aldosterone levels in obese patients. *New England Journal of Medicine, 304,* 930.

Tucker, K. L., Mahnken, B., Wilson, P. W., Jacques, P., & Selhub, J. (1996). Folic acid fortification of the food supply. Potential benefits and risks for the elderly population. *Journal of the American Medical Association, 276,* 1879-1885.

Turner, R. T., Riggs, B. L., & Spelsberg, T. C. (1994). Skeletal effects of estrogen. *Endocrine Review, 15,* 275-300.

Udoff, L., Langenberg, P., & Adashi, E. Y. (1995). Combined continuous hormone replacement therapy: A critical review. *Obstetrics & Gynecology, 86,* 306-316.

Urinary Incontinence Guideline Panel. (1992). *Urinary incontinence in adults: Clinical practice guideline* (AHCRR Publication No. 92-0038). Rockville, MD: Agency for Health Care Policy and Research, Public Health Service, U.S. Department of Health and Human Services.

U.S. Department of Health and Human Services. (1988). *Surgeon General's report on nutrition and health.* Washington, DC: Government Printing Office.

U.S. Department of Health and Human Services. (1991). *Healthy people 2000: National health promotion and disease prevention objectives* (DHSS Publication No. PHS-91-50212). Washington DC: Government Printing Office.

U.S. Department of Health and Human Services. (1996). *Physical activity and health: A report of the Surgeon General.* Alanta, GA: USDHHS, Centers for Disease Control and Prevention, National Center for Chronic Disease Prevention and Health Promotion.

Valdez, R., Seidell, J. C., Ahn, Y. L., & Weiss, K. M. (1993). A new index of abdominal adiposity as an indicator for cardiovascular disease. A cross-population study. *International Journal of Obesity, 17*(2), 77-82.

van der Kooy, K., & Seidell, J. C. (1993). Techniques for the measurement of visceral fat: A practical guide. *International Journal of Obesity and Related Metabolic Disorders, 17,* 187-196.

Vandervoort, A. A., Chesworth, B. M., Cunningham, D. A., Rechnitzer, R. A., Paterson, D. H., & Koval, J. J. (1992). An outcome measure to quantify passive stiffness of the ankle. *Canadian Journal of Public Health, 83*(Suppl. 2), 519-523.

Van Poppel, G., & Goldbohm, R. A. (1995). Epidemiologic evidence for beta-carotene and cancer prevention. *American Journal of Clinical Nutrition, 62,* 1393S-1402S.

Verbrugge, L. M. (1989). The dynamics of population aging and health. In S. J. Lewis (Ed.), *Aging and health: Linking research and public policy* (pp. 23-40). Chelsea, MI: Lewis.

Verdeal, K., & Ryan, D. (1979). Naturally-occurring estrogens in plant foodstuffs: A review. *Journal of Food Protein, 42,* 577-583.

Verhoef, P., Stampfer, M. J., & Rimm, E. B. (1998). Folate and coronary heart disease. *Current Opinion of Lipidology, 9*(1), 17-22.

Vestal, R. E. (1990). Clinical pharmacology. In W. R. Hazzard, R. Andres, E. L. Bierman, & J. P. Blass (Eds.), *Principles of geriatric medicine and gerontology* (2nd ed., pp. 201-211). New York: McGraw-Hill.

Vestal, R. E., & Dawson, G. W. (1985). Pharmacology and aging. In C. E. Finch & E. L. Schneider (Eds.), *Handbook of the biology of aging* (2nd ed., pp. 744-819). New York: Van Nostrand Rienhold.

Vokonas, P. S., & Kannel, W. B. (1996). Risk factors for and prevention of atherosclerotic cardiovascular disease. In J. S. Alpert (Ed.), *Cardiology for the primary care physician* (pp. 89-98). St. Louis, MO: C. V. Mosby.

Vokonas, P. S., Kannel, W. B., & Cupples, L. A. (1988). Epidemiology and risk of hypertension in the elderly: The Framingham Study. *Journal of Hypertension, 6*(Suppl.), 3-9.

Voorrips, L. E., Lemmink, K. A. P. M., Van Heuvelen, M. J. G., Bult, P., & Van Staveren, W. A. (1993). The physical conditioning of elderly women differing in habitual physical activity. *Medicine and Science in Sports and Exercise, 23,* 1152-1157.

Wagner, J. D., Clarkson, T. B., St. Clair, R. W., Schwenke, D. C., Shively, C. A., & Adams, M. R. (1991). Estrogen and progesterone replacement therapy reduces low density lipoprotein accumulation in the coronary arteries of surgically postmenopausal cynomolgus monkeys. *Journal of Clinical Investigations, 88,* 1995-2002.

Wallerstein, N. (1992). Powerlessness, empowerment, and health implications for health promotion programs. *American Journal of Health Promotion, 6,* 149-170.

Wallerstein, N., & Bernstein, E. (1994). Introduction to community empowerment, participatory education and health. *Health Education Quarterly, 21,* 141-148.

Wamala, S. P., Wolk, A., Schenck-Gustafsson, K., & Orth-Gomer, K. (1997). Lipid profile and socioeconomic status in healthy middle aged women in Sweden. *Journal of Epidemiology and Community Health, 51,* 400-407.

Wang, Q., Hassager, C., Ravn, P., Wang, S., & Christiansen, C. (1994). Total and regional body-composition changes in early postmenopausal women: Age-related or menopause-related? *American Journal of Clinical Nutrition, 60,* 843-848.

Warner, K. E., Slade, J., & Sweanor, D. T. (1997). The emerging market for long-term nicotine maintenance. *Journal of the American Medical Association, 278,* 1087-1092.

Weber, P., Bendich, A., & Machlin, L. J. (1997). Vitamin E and human health: Rationale for determining recommended intake levels. *Nutrition, 13,* 450-460.

Webster, J. R., & Cain, T. (1997). Pulmonary disease. In C. K. Cassel, H. J. Cohen, E. B. Larson, D. E. Meier, N. M. Resnick, L. Z. Rubenstein, & L. B. Sorensen (Eds.), *Geriatric medicine* (3rd ed., pp. 653-665). New York: Springer.

Wei, J. Y., & Gersh, B. J. (1987). Heart disease in the elderly. *Current Problems of Cardiology, 12*(1), 1-65.

Weinberg, A. D., & Minaker, K. L. (1995). Dehydration: Evaluation and management in elder adults (Council on Scientific Affairs, American Medical Association). *Journal of the American Medical Association 25,* 2249-2254.

Weindruch, R., & Sohal, R. S. (1997). Seminars in medicine of the Beth Israel Deaconess Medical Center: Caloric intake and aging. *New England Journal of Medicine, 337,* 986-994.

Weiss, N. S. (1996). Health consequences of short- and long-term postmenopausal hormone therapy. *Clinical Chemistry, 42*(8, Pt. 2), 1342-1344.

Weiss, R. (1989). Reflections on the present state of loneliness research. In M. Hojat & R. Crandall (Eds.), *Loneliness: Theory, research and applications* (pp. 1-16). Newbury Park, CA: Sage.

Wenger, N. K. (1993). Coronary heart disease: Diagnostic decision making. In P. S. Douglas (Ed.), *Heart disease in women* (pp. 3-21). Philadelphia: W. B. Saunders.

Wenger, N. K. (1997). Cardiovascular disease. In C. K. Cassel, H. J. Cohen, E. B. Larson, D. E. Meier, N. M. Resnick, L. Z. Rubenstein, & L. B. Sorensen (Eds.), *Geriatric medicine* (3rd ed., pp. 357-389). New York: Springer.

Wenger, N. K., O'Rourke, R. A., & Marcus, F. I. (1988). The care of elderly patients with cardiovascular disease. *Annals of Internal Medicine, 109,* 425-428.

Wetter, D. W., Fiore, M. C., Gritz, E. R., Lando, H. A., Stitzer, M. L., Hasselblad, V., & Baker, T. B. (1998). The Agency for Health Care Policy and Research smoking cessation clinical practice guideline: Findings and implications for psychologists. *American Psychology, 53,* 657-669.

Whited, J. D., Hall, R. P., Russell, P., Simel, D. L., & Horner, R. D. (1997). Primary care clinicians' performance for detecting actinic keratoses and skin cancer. *Archives of Internal Medicine, 157,* 985-990.

Willcox, S. M., Himmelstein, D. U., & Woolhandler, S. (1994). Inappropriate drug prescribing for the community-dwelling elderly. *Journal of the American Medical Association, 272,* 292-296.

Willett, W. C., Green, A., Stampfer, M. J., Speizer, F. E., Colditz, G. A., Rosner, B., Monson, R. R., Stason, W., & Hennekens, C. H. (1987). Relative and absolute excess risks of coronary heart disease among women who smoke cigarettes. *New England Journal of Medicine, 317,* 1303-1309.

Williams, J. E., & Flora, J. A. (1995). Health behavior segmentation and campaign planning to reduce cardiovascular disease risk among Hispanics. *Health Education Quarterly, 22*(1), 36-48.

Williams, M. A. (1994). *Exercise testing and training in the elderly cardiac patient.* Champaign, IL: Human Kinetics.

Williams, R. B. (1987). Refine the type-A hypothesis: Emergence of the hostility complex. *American Journal of Cardiology, 60,* 27J-32J.

Williams, R. R., Hunt, S. C., Hasstedt, S. J., Hopkins, P. N., Wu, L. L., Berry, T. D., Stults, B. M., Barlow, G. K., & Kuida, H. (1990). Genetics of hypertension: What we know and don't know. *Clinical & Experimental Hypertension—Part A, Theory & Practice, 12,* 865-876.

Wing, R. R., Matthews, K. A., Kuller, L. H., Meilahn, E. N., & Plantinga, P. (1991). Waist to hip ratio in middle aged women: Associations with behavioral and psychosocial factors with changes in cardiovascular risk factors. *Arteriosclerosis and Thrombosis, 11,* 1250-1257.

Wing, S., Casper, M., Riggan, W., Hayes, C., & Tyroler, H. A. (1988). Socioenvironmental characteristics associated with the onset of decline of ischemic heart disease mortality in the United States. *American Journal of Public Health, 78,* 923-926.

Wolfe, R., Morrow, J., & Fredrickson, B. L. (1996). Mood disorders in older adults. In L. L. Carstensen, B. A. Edelstein, & L. Dornbrand (Eds.), *The practical handbook of clinical gerontology* (pp. 274-303). Thousand Oaks, CA: Sage.

Wood, P. D., Stefanick, M. L., Williams, P. T., & Haskell, W. L. (1991). The effects on plasma lipoproteins of a prudent weight-reducing diet, with or without exercise, in overweight men and women. *New England Journal of Medicine, 325,* 461-466.

Woollacott, M. H. (1993). Age-related changes in posture and movement. *Journal of Gerontology, 48,* 56-60.

Young, V. D., Munro, H. N., & Fukayama, N. (1989). Protein and functional consequences of deficiency in nutrition in the elderly. In H. Horowitz, D. A. MacFadgen, H. Munro, et al. (Eds.), *Motivation in the elderly.* Oxford, UK: Oxford University Press.

Zemel, M. B., Zemel, P. C., Bryg, R. J., & Sowers, J. R. (1990). Dietary calcium induces regression of left ventricular hypertrophy in hypertensive non-insulin-dependent diabetic blacks. *American Journal of Hypertension, 3*(6, Pt. 1), 458-463.

Zheng, W., Doyle, T., Kushi, L., Sellers, T., Hong, C., & Folsom, A. (1996). Tea consumption and cancer incidence in a prospective cohort study of postmenopausal women. *American Journal of Epidemiology, 144,* 175-182.

Index

About the Authors

Colleen Keller, R.N., PhD, is Professor in the Department of Family Care Nursing at the University of Texas Health Sciences Center at San Antonio. Her research has focused on reduction of cardiovascular risk factors in women of diverse ethnic backgrounds, with an emphasis on obesity and sedentary activity as particular risk behaviors. She has received funding from the American Heart Association, Sigma Theta Tau, and the American Nurses' Foundation. Keller maintains a clinical practice at an inner-city clinic, providing primary care to underserved individuals. She has participated on national committees for the American Heart Association's Council on Cardiovascular Nursing and the American Academy of Nurse Practitioners.

Julie Fleury, R.N., PhD, is Associate Professor in the Department of Adult and Geriatric Health at the University of North Carolina at Chapel Hill. Her research has included development and refinement of the middle range wellness motivation theory, instrument development and testing, and the creation and testing of theory-based interventions designed to promote secondary prevention of cardiovascular disease. Much of her work has focused on the cultural and contextual relevance of motivational concepts and measures, particularly in older, underserved populations. Her recently funded NINR/National Institutes of Health study, "Motivation in the Maintenance of Physical Activity," is a multisite, community-based study that includes as predictors of regular physical activity evaluation of cultural context, self-knowledge in goal formation, the appraisal of readiness, and self-regulation. Fleury currently serves as codirector for the Intervention Core of the Center for Research on Chronic Illness at the School of Nursing, University of North Carolina at Chapel Hill. She has participated on national committees for the American Association of Critical Care Nursing, Sigma Theta Tau International, and the American Heart Association's Council on Cardiovascular Nursing.